ANSWERS IN THE HEART

ANSWERS IN THE HEART

DAILY MEDITATIONS
FOR MEN AND WOMEN
RECOVERING FROM SEX ADDICTION

HazelDeN®

First published October 1989.

ISBN-13: 978-0-89486-568-8
ISBN-10: 0-89486-568-4
Library of Congress Catalog Card Number: 89-83560
Printed in the United States of America.

This book is dedicated
to the men and women in
my recovery group who
are the voices of this book.

PW

Editor's note: The authors, a man and a woman, have chosen to remain anonymous. Authorship is indicated by the distinctive ligatures, PW and SK, at the end of each meditation.

INTRODUCTION

Sex addiction is a betrayal of the loving heart. Like all addictions, it is cunning, baffling, powerful—and destructive. It often has its roots in childhood in unhealthy family relationships where there was boundary trespassing, seduction, violence, and other abuse. Sex addiction then may continue in secrecy from generation to generation. Those of us who were abused often kept seeking out situations that seemed to promise gratification, but that inevitably brought humiliation and pain. We tried to figure out the obscure mechanism that drove our behavior, and we may have even managed to work out some kind of explanation. But more often than not, we continued acting out and reenacting our desperate scenarios. Our behavior remained inexplicable, implacable, and devastating.

To understand what was happening to us, we found we needed to change the beliefs that underlaid and motivated our behavior. What we discovered continues to be true at each stage of our recovery: We need to be honest, fearless, and confront our affliction by breaking out of our secrets and shame. Above all, we need to develop new ways of interpreting our feelings and expressing them, and new ways of loving and relating to the world.

Love is the antidote to addiction. By love, we mean the abiding affection that comes from connecting with others. This love includes and nurtures our sexuality as we rethink the relationship between love and power. Such love does not exist in isolation, and so we are moved toward other men and women to find and develop it.

Most of us were enslaved by our addiction as long as we were convinced that we were unlovable and therefore incapable of loving others. For many of us, our search brought us to Twelve Step programs that offer vital and nurturing communities where we can learn the simple truths of loving and allowing ourselves to be loved. It is here we can find the serenity and strength to daily turn our struggles over to a Power greater than ourselves. Often, spiritual healing brought sexual healing as we recognized and expressed ourselves as whole people, with both masculine and feminine aspects. In these programs we continue to find confidence and fellowship as we open ourselves to others and our Higher Power. We begin to feel at ease, at home in a community.

It is our hope that these meditations will also bring the reader to a wider community. In writing them, we've tried to give voices to people who have known the suffering, loneliness, and shame of sex addiction, and yet did not abandon hope or turn against life. They, perhaps like you, have begun to find new hope and life in recovery.

May they speak through us to you, from heart to heart.

January

*Lift us, we pray thee, to thy presence, where
we may be still and know that thou art God.*
— Book of Common Prayer

Solitude carries with it a risk, and the risk is loneliness. It is as if we are in the center of a city, then decide to leave. As we travel toward the suburbs, there are fewer and fewer people. Finally, the city is behind us, and we are alone. And since we cannot live in two places at once, we attain the pleasure of solitude and pay the price of loneliness.

It is the same when we leave behind the noise of our own thoughts and travel inward. It takes courage to face solitude, a courage which our Higher Power will give us when we want to find what we cannot find when we are surrounded by people. Peace, inspiration, rejuvenation, nurturing, enlightenment, strength — these are the gifts of solitude.

Beyond the loneliness, and the longing for others, we find the satisfaction of our own company and the company of God. We need these as much as we need the company of people, and so we will receive what we need to take the risks of solitude.

---

*There is nothing to fear in solitude. I may feel alone, but
I never am.*

SK

Where is there dignity unless there is honesty?
— *Cicero*

In our program of recovery, nothing is more precious and productive than honesty. Our sex addiction made us secretive and devious, and warped our judgment. Many of us may have even taken perverse pleasure in leading a double life, though we ended up deceiving and hurting ourselves above all.

We are reclaiming our integrity and our honor. We are begining to feel worthy of love and affection, as we learn to give affection and love to others.

Our program bids us to make "a searching and fearless moral inventory of ourselves." Without rigorous honesty, such a step is impossible — but without completing this task, our program will lead nowhere. Only if we are honest can we move toward the truth of ourselves and regain our dignity. At first it will be painful, but each day and each step along the way moves us forward, toward the power of openness and integrity.

Honesty is hard for me, but I am learning to think and speak fearlessly about my addiction and its crippling effects on my life.

PW

*God, why do I storm heaven for answers that
are already in my heart? Every grace I need
has already been given me. Oh, lead me to the
Beyond within.*

— *Macrina Wiederkehr*

Once we were abstinent, it was overwhelming to find
out all the feelings our sex addiction covered up. Maybe
they were frozen or pushed down. Maybe they became
distorted, such as unexpressed anger that turns into self-
righteousness. Maybe we don't even know how we feel
or we can't name our feelings. It's difficult to let ourselves feel, especially when the feelings are connected
to a past trauma like childhood sexual abuse or incest.
It's also painful to relive feelings we had when we were
practicing our addiction. But it's necessary.

There's no joy without sorrow; our feelings cannot
be neatly compartmentalized and controlled. To know
how we feel is to add real richness to our lives. It's to
see in color what we've been seeing in black-and-white.
Our feelings are the basis for our reality and our actions.

*Humbly asking my Higher Power to remove my shortcom-
ings helps restore my feelings by restoring my sense of myself.*

SK

*I like the dreams of the future better than the
history of the past.*
— *Thomas Jefferson*

Our past is already in place and nothing can change
it. Yet we do keep on reinterpreting it, and that is wise,
since our present attitudes can be renewed by relating
them to our past experiences. Often, especially with our
families and friends, we never cease revising our in-
terpretations and evaluations of the past; we need to
keep doing this so that we can live fully and freely.

Only when we have the past in some kind of healthy
perspective can we live richly in the present and dream
of the future. Then our lives open up a space for ex-
perimentation and play.

We need our dreams and should cherish them, but
they will come to us more freely when we are comfortable with our past. Working the Twelve Steps allows us
to share our feelings about the past and build dreams
as we are on our path of recovery.

*I know that I must understand my past before the future
can be truly a place of dreams.*

PW

*Shame is the motor behind compulsive be-
havior.*

— *Anonymous*

Shame. Even the word is stark. When we feel shame,
we feel utterly worthless, not because of what we've
done, but because of who we think we are. We think
we are unlovable, incapable of giving love. The more our
addiction progressed, the more out of control and
powerless we felt. That's when we found shame waiting in the chaos. We wanted to be invisible, to disappear.

But there was something we wanted more: a way out.
We found it by hanging on to the knowledge that we
have dignity because we have life. It was given to us by
our Higher Power who loves us unconditionally. We no
longer need to feel shame because we no longer need
to use people or let ourselves be used. Instead, we live
in the grace and light of recovery, with dignity and in
peace.

---

*What counteracts shame? Honesty about my feelings, bound-
aries, living in the present, getting out of my self-absorption.
These are how I can take care of myself. Above all, gentleness and self-forgiveness will restore my emotional balance.*

SK

A child miseducated is a child lost.
— *John F. Kennedy*

So much money is spent on bombs and missiles and so little on education. With so many children still in crowded classrooms and old buildings, with ill-trained and ill-paid teachers, it seems easier for us to destroy life than to nurture and strengthen it.

What was it like for us as children? "Education" means leading out from...away from ignorance, defenselessness, anxiety, and fear. Were we educated in this sense, or were we neglected or even abused?

Childhood especially should be a time of growth and hope. When memories of childhood are tarnished, bitterness and resentment follow, and these in turn can lead to erratic or addictive behavior. As sex addicts, we know what it was like to be pushed away, exploited, even seduced or abused. We hated it and it made us distrustful and angry.

Now, in recovery, we feel the power of "education" as we learn to leave behind the ignorance, fear, and pain of our childhood. We come to feel the joy of nurturing ourselves and caring deeply for those around us.

I want to be concerned with education as a way of overcoming ignorance, mistrust, isolation, and fear.

PW

*Most people write off their longing for friends
and family as so many losses in their lives,
when they should count the fact that their heart
is able to long so hard and to love so much
as among their greatest blessings.*
— Etty Hillesum

It was lonely being a practicing sex addict. When we
were being sexual with someone else, we could push
the truth away for a while in the high of the moment.
But afterward, back in reality, the loneliness became even
more devastating. We could pretend not to care, telling
ourselves that we didn't need people. But we knew we
were lying. Connection, not disconnection, was what
we longed for.

It's possible to rebuild the connections we lost to our
addiction. But even in recovery, the loneliness doesn't
go away immediately; it takes time. The more we reach
out to people honestly, believing we are worthwhile and
have something to give, the less lonely we feel. There's
a world out there, and we belong in it.

*Who am I lonely for? God? Myself? Other people? Once
I answer that, I can do something about it.*

SK

*An old error is always more popular than a
new truth.*

— German proverb

We often feel uncomfortable with the new because
it causes us to reach out and expand our vision. This
may be painful and we don't like the pain that comes
with change and recovery.

Our sex addiction was cozy and gave us a curious kind
of comfort and reassurance. We turned to it when we
were lonely or anxious or hopeless. We were used to
it and didn't need to do much to keep on going in the
same old way.

Suddenly, we saw the error of our ways. Discovery,
disgrace, a suit for damages, prison, isolation, despair,
the loss of a spouse, the contempt of our friends — are
all possible consequences of that cozy old addiction.
Yes, we may have awakened one day to find that our
addiction had ruined our lives. We began then reaching out for the hard process of change.

Making difficult changes is painful, but that pain is
far preferable to the agony caused by the inevitable outcome of our addiction.

---

*I am reaching and embracing the new even though it is
sometimes painful for a while.*

PW

Out of suffering have emerged the strongest souls; the most massive characters are seared with scars.

— *E. H. Chapin*

When we are suffering, what do we do with it? Do we use it as a reason to abuse ourselves, shame ourselves, or hate ourselves? Do we turn to our sex addiction to escape from the pain that is part of suffering?

When we were acting out, we suffered, we felt pain, but we usually didn't understand why. The suffering and pain that accompanies recovery is different — it leads to healing, or it will if we let it. Sometimes we can turn our pain over to our Higher Power, trusting that our pain is there to help us grow, and that it will pass. This can help us believe that our pain has a purpose.

Our feelings, no matter how difficult some of them are to feel, are supported by the compassion we're learning to feel for ourselves and the compassion God feels for us.

I can choose to look at my pain in the light of recovery. It won't last forever; I will survive.

SK

And nothing to look backward to with pride,
And nothing to look forward to with hope.
— *Robert Frost*

Sex addiction is an illness that can easily lead us to lose our pride and hope. Often our lives seem poisoned at the very source. We can't remember a time of innocence, joy, or confidence in ourselves and our relationships with others. Perhaps we were sexually or verbally abused as children. We may feel unsure of our boundaries, and view the future with anxiety and dread. Will nothing ever change?

To go forward we have to admit that we are powerless to undo the hurt and abuse of the past. And we learn that we can no longer go it alone; we have been alone too long. The first two Steps of our program help us overcome the past and turn toward the future with growing hope and trust. And then the present, like the New Year, becomes filled with promise.

By accepting that our lives have been unmanageable and by turning to our Higher Power, we find new pride and hope in our daily lives.

PW

Our first priority must be our individual recovery; only when we have succeeded in improving our self-esteem will we be able to be in a relationship truly by choice and not out of dependency.

— *Jennifer and Burt Schneider*

Sex is not glue. It doesn't keep people with us. We've often misunderstood sexuality and intimacy when we were active in our addiction because our addiction distorted our experiences.

Finding the way to real intimacy with ourselves, friends, a significant other, or our family is difficult. But we know that real intimacy is a connection that is natural.

It takes self-esteem to know that someone loves us for ourselves and wants to be with us just because we are who we are. There's no way we can control our relationships, especially a relationship intimate enough to be sexual. We just have to let go and trust. That's true freedom.

I am always a sexual being, whether I choose to express my sexuality or not. The energy and goodness of my sexuality are my unique gift from God.

SK

*I'd never seen men hold each other. I thought
the only thing they were allowed to do was
shake hands or fight.*

— Rita Mae Brown

Many of us, perhaps men more than women, have
grown up without knowing the warmth of lovingly
touching one another. Some of us had fathers who
trapped themselves in a stereotypical male role, afraid
to hold us and show their love for us. We may have
learned to be independent, competitive, and separate.
We often fell into awkwardness and isolation. As men
especially, we became afraid to reach out, hug, and hold
someone of our own sex.

Whether male or female, so many of us have lost touch
with ourselves and with others. We have been alone
too long.

One of the really healthy things about many Twelve
Step meetings is the custom of holding one another and
giving hugs. At first we may find it embarrassing and keep
our distance. But as we learn to loosen up and reach out,
we look forward to the warmth and strength that comes
from giving and receiving a friendly, caring hug. It is
good to learn to touch in a fearless and nonsexual way.

*I am glad to be in touch with other people through hugging
and holding.*

PW

*Humankind owes to the child the best it has
to give.*
— *United Nations Declaration*

We need to be committed to recovery for ourselves,
but there may be others in our lives for whom our
recovery is also vital: our children, for example. The
Twelve Step program's wisdom says that our children
start recovering the same day we do. No matter what
our family's past has been, when we recover, we know
we have broken the cycle of addiction not only for ourselves, but for the children we cherish.

Our children can grow up healthy, with the Twelve
Step program to guide and educate them in the realities of addiction. They'll have a greater opportunity to
flourish in the love and new way of life we are learning.
To see them serene and reaching their potential can be
one of the happiest gifts of our recovery.

---

*God, with Your help, my children will shine like the sun.
Please hold them today in the palm of Your hand.*

SK

It is better to be hated for what you are than loved for what you are not.

— *Andre Gide*

If we live with someone we really love and betray the person with our sex addiction, we are living a lie. More and more, we shun intimacy and turn toward our distorted world.

But what of our loved ones? The persons we are deceiving may begin doubting us and end up feeling crazy. Deception, half-truths, missed appointments, financial irresponsibility, loss of job, lies, and more lies — all turn a loving relationship into a twisted nightmare. There seems to be no way out.

One single Step, the First Step in our program, and the journey toward recovery begins. We begin to learn how to be honest and to look people in the eye again. We come to own our actions and face our loved ones. At first, our journey will be painful, but with love and patience and trust we will come through.

In overcoming my sex addiction I will regain the love and trust of my loved ones.

PW

This cup holds grief and balm in equal measure. Light, darkness. Who drinks from it must change.

— May Sarton

"This addiction hurts so much," one recovering person used to say. As sex addicts, we understand how she feels. Our struggle to give up abusive sexual practices or relationships is often difficult and can seem overwhelming at times. Yet, we're doing the asking; we're challenging ourselves to change. We must never give up hope. We must hang on, even when it's so hard we don't know how we're doing it. Living a day, even an hour, at a time can help us make it through.

We're not alone. We have our Higher Power. We have the support of our group, with all the love and understanding they so freely share. We have the Twelve Steps and our daily program. Most of all, we have our abstinence and our willingness. Even if the abstinence is only a few days and our willingness is only a shred, that's enough.

To be in recovery is to be willing to go to any lengths. I know I can do it.

SK

I am a part of all that I have met.
— *Alfred Tennyson*

Too often we lose our way by forgetting that we are part of a community, a society, a world. When we were in our addiction, we closed ourselves off from others and drifted along alone. Fantasy, rituals, and acting out took us not out of ourselves, but deeper into loneliness.

As we go through life we make contact with others even if we don't always realize it. Looking, talking, smiling, touching, eating, walking, working, playing — all these activities are likely to bring us into contact with others. And the way we act and react does make a difference. Often a simple smile can make someone else's day. A hug breaks the ice of solitude. A kind word strikes a chord and is remembered.

Yes, we are part of humanity and we get love and power from knowing this.

I want to feel part of a community of people in recovery.

PW

If today you hear God's voice, harden not your hearts.

— Ps. 95:7-8

Sometimes it seems as though our obsession with sex will never go away. The fantasies, the secret longings, the compulsion triggered by a song, a movie, a look seem so deeply rooted within us. We sometimes can't imagine living without our addiction, no matter how much we want to.

Yet, we've met people in recovery who are free from their obsessive preoccupation with sex. It may happen suddenly or it may take years, but our faith in recovery tells us it will happen. We're on our path, and we get all the time we need. All we have to do today is be willing and make the best choices we can. That's where our Higher Power comes in.

Perhaps we hear exactly what we need to hear in our recovery group. A friend may call, just when we think that no one really cares. Or, it may simply be those moments of peace we experience as prayer and meditation become a genuine part of our daily lives. Gradually, we realize that freedom was there all the time, a gift that's ours as soon as we're willing to accept it.

God can do the impossible. I know God is stronger than my addiction.

SK

Sex is one of the nine reasons for reincarnation. The other eight are unimportant.
— Henry Miller

It is good and healthy to laugh about sex — as long as the laughter is on the side of life. Sex, after all, is part of the life force, and if it is surrounded by caring and honesty, it leads to a joyous intensification of our relationship with others and with the world. Then sex, like laughter, integrates.

Too often laughing about sex betrays uneasiness, shame, disgust, and the desire to hurt. We talk about "dirty jokes" and consign sex to the bathroom. We split off sex from other feelings and surround it with taboos and rituals and mockery. Viewed in this way, sex isolates us.

We need to learn to talk about our sexuality in a proud and affirmative way. Talking and laughing in a group, or with a friend, or with a loved one, is one of the steps we take to bring sex into the open to take its place as a part of the diversity of life.

I want to own my sexuality, to talk about it without shame, and to claim it as a vital part of my life.

PW

Courage is fear that has said its prayers.
— One Day at a Time in Al-Anon

Nothing freezes us in our tracks like fear. How many times have we let fear stop us from doing what we really wanted to do? Maybe we wanted to look for a job, be honest with a friend, ask someone for a date, buy a house. But we couldn't because we were afraid. The truth is, the moment our fear takes control, our self-will also takes control.

The first thing to do is to admit to ourselves that we're afraid. The second is to find out why. Discovering why may mean calling a friend to talk, praying, taking an inventory of ourselves, going to a meeting. To feel the fear lift is to have ourselves back again. Then, when we know how we feel, we'll know what to do.

Can I accept my Higher Power's help and the help of others when I'm afraid? Emotional balance and serenity unclouded by fear are the gifts of recovery.

SK

A merry heart doeth good like a medicine.
— *Prov. 17:22*

When we are gloomy and melancholy we seem to walk around in a black cloud. We attract other disheartened people to us, and soon it seems as if we are marching along in a funeral procession.

To be permanently gloomy seems an insult to life. After all, there are many people who are worse off than we, and yet they manage to find the energy and love to reach out and express joy. Why should we be in the gloomy minority?

Often it is our addiction that dictates our moods. When we were acting out we led a double life with half of it rooted in shame and fear. It's no wonder that we were down, and that we sometimes carry this habit and attitude into our recovery.

Part of recovery is regaining a sense of happiness that reaches into the deepest part of us. We can hear ourselves laugh again and learn to play. What a tonic it is to be happy!

Joy is a vital part of life and I want to feel it deep inside me.

PW

We seek God until He finds us.
— Madeleine L'Engle

The day comes when we suddenly realize we are not caught up in our addiction. That's the moment we know we're living in recovery, that we're practicing the principles of recovery in all areas of our lives.

This awakening can come suddenly, as the result of a crisis, or it can happen subtly, over time. It always brings with it a deepening of our commitment to the Twelve Step program. We find ourselves turning away from the addiction and toward our Higher Power. We find the joy of living in God's will.

Working the Twelve Steps frees us from the tyranny of sex addiction by giving us the awareness that God has removed the addiction because we've let go of it. Things are restored to their proper order. The addiction is outside of us; we have ourselves and our relationship with our Higher Power. It's then that we can reach out to other sex addicts because we finally have someone to give them — ourselves.

I am not my addiction. My addiction is not my Higher Power.

SK

What are we faced with in the nineteenth century? An age where Woman was sacred and where you could buy a thirteen-year-old girl for a few pounds.

— *John Fowles*

There is often a double standard in men's attitude to women. Men idealize women, perhaps on the basis of their love for their mothers, and yet they exploit and debase them in pornography and prostitution.

Sex addiction increases this split. Men who are sex addicts place women up high on pedestals, and at the same time break down their real identity into images and fragments in pornographic pictures. They relate to women not for affection and caring, but to appease their anonymous lusts.

To be human means to have our faults and virtues. To allow people to be real allows emotions. Then, there can be real respect and love that doesn't need to idealize beyond reality or debase to the lowest depths.

In our recovery we gain a new perspective on our attitudes and conduct toward all our fellow human beings.

I am learning to treat all other people not as objects of selfish gratification but as dignified and beautiful children of the universe.

PW

I am a glorious being. A miracle. That which is in God is also in me. I survive all the storms, and like a tree planted by the water, I shall not be moved.

— *Susan L. Taylor*

Sex addiction is a spiritual disease. Yes, our mind, body, and emotions were affected, but in the end, it was our spirit that was most deeply wounded. That's because of the wondrous, vulnerable link between our sexuality and our spirit.

Despite the trauma of our addiction, despite the battering our spirit took, it was never broken. Some part of us stayed safe until we could be led toward healing.

Who we are transcends human understanding. The knowledge of who we are can only be experienced by the heart, glimpsed occasionally with joy and humility as our recovery progresses. We are thankful that some part of us was kept safe, waiting for our recovery. "We are walking miracles," said one group member. We are.

To be true to my own spirit is to say yes to God's will and to life itself.

SK

When the fight begins within himself
A man's worth something.
— *Robert Browning*

Sex addiction is a powerful disease that knocks the stuffing out of us. When our lives are controlled by it, by our obsessions and compulsions about sex, we don't seem to have much energy — or courage, or hope — left for the rest of life. We are driven back into ourselves and we lack the energy to come out and participate in life.

This is the power of sex addiction. Many of us spent hours seeking opportunities to act out or get lost in our fantasies. We fought and fought these desires, but we eventually tired. We may have even wanted to stop struggling against our addiction and let it take us over and ruin our lives.

Getting into a program is the recognition that we mean to put up a fight on different terms. We are tired of being sick and tired; we need a new power base; we want to act from real strength. Looking around, we see men and women on the move, actively choosing to turn their struggle with their addiction over to their Higher Power. We join them and feel our energies renewed and we see hope along the open road.

I'm tired of being defeated by my addiction; I want to join with others in turning over the struggle and be free.

PW

If the will remains in protest, it stays dependent on that which it is protesting against. If apathy is to be avoided in such paralysis of the will, the individual needs to ask, "Is there something in me that is a cause of, or contributes to, my paralysis?"

— *Rollo May*

Trusting only our will is one of the characteristics of addiction. In our addiction, we used our will in a misguided way to try to deny the past or even change it. We used our will to try to control ourselves and others. Willpower, as such, has no place in recovery. Working a Twelve Step program helps us change the way we use our will.

The more we realize that a Higher Power's will is operating in our lives, the more we can use our will as it should be used—to make the efforts necessary to carry out God's will for us. This takes us out of the past and into the present. Facing the past honestly, rather than applying our will to reinforce our version of the past, puts us firmly in the present, living today only.

The past is over. I will find God's will for me in what happens to me today.

SK

[Man] thinks of himself as a creator instead of a user, and this delusion is robbing him of the earth.

— *Helen Hoover*

Sometimes, in our grandiose view of ourselves and our world, we think we have all the time and space we want to do our will. But in reality, our resources are limited, and already we are losing needed material and precious species that will never return to our planet.

Let us remember we are here only for a short while, but others will come after us. We need to take care of our earth just as much as we need to take care of ourselves. If we think only of our own pleasure, we are likely to become selfish and live destructive lives.

Those of us who are sex addicts realize how much we squandered our energy and dissipated vital forces. We tried to impose our fantasies and our wills on other people and we abused those who needed our love and trust. We thought we were little gods and that the world was here just for us. Now, in recovery, we can learn to take care of ourselves and the world that surrounds us.

It is good to be aware of all that is precious in our world, including ourselves.

PW

It is a true proverb, that if you live with a lame man you will learn to halt.

— *Plutarch*

Working through the memories of childhood is a task each of us eventually faces. Just as an alcoholic family system contributes to alcoholism, so too does a family addicted to sex affect our addiction as adults.

We can decide whether it's important for us to know if and how sex addiction has operated in our families. We can gain that knowledge as we need it. But simply knowing that the addiction is real, that it's present in family systems, and that we didn't cause it helps us to stop blaming ourselves.

The important thing is to concentrate on our own recovery. We cannot change our families or the past, but we can change our attitudes toward them. When we feel caught up in a family member's addictive behavior, we can bring our attention back to ourselves. That way, resentment and fruitless anger yield to honesty and humility. Detaching from the things we cannot change, forgiving the harm done to us, and letting go of the past are important parts of our healing.

Just for today, I will let go of anger and resentment toward my family and focus on taking care of myself.

SK

If Winter comes
Can Spring be far behind?
— *Percy Bysshe Shelley*

We do not need to be afraid of winter. In winter nature lies fallow in preparation for the new year. All life needs rest in order to grow with greater strength, and winter is the time of withdrawal that precedes renewal.

Sometimes it may seem that our lives have become dark and hopeless and we can't see a way forward. Perhaps a relationship has gone sour and we think it must be the end. Work goes badly; money is a problem; our children go away. We become lost in our melancholy and feel things will never get better.

We can draw strength from the wisdom of the seasons. Bare trees will become clothed in green, and the hard earth will again yield harvests of plenty. We can appreciate this transformation as it happens every year, and we can take hope from it. We can also see our lives as bound to change.

Nothing in my life need defeat me, since I know that spring and summer will always come again.

PW

I will not fear, for you are ever with me, and
you will never leave me to face my perils alone.
— *Thomas Merton*

When we're struggling with our addiction, then is the
time to remember that we can't have it both ways. We
can't assume that because something in our life is hard,
we're free to turn to our addiction to retreat from reality.
The addiction may pull us, but it's only a pull. It's nothing more than a pull until we choose to act on it.

Stop here to remember the insanity of the thinking
we have used to justify acting out. Remember too that
there is a Power greater than ourselves who will relieve
our suffering and the pressure of our addiction. What
a relief to know we're not alone. There is hope. We can
have peace, abstinence, and the happy life of recovery
— or we can have the well-remembered horrors of
our addiction. It's not always an easy choice, but it is
our choice.

I am able to see clearly the consequences of the choices
I make. I choose recovery.

SK

A mighty flame follows a tiny spark.
— *Dante*

It is hard for many of us to say how and when we became addicted to destructive sexual acting out. At first, we may have been under the influence of alcohol or other drugs or perhaps we acted out of anger or despair. It might have been only a tiny slip or push that started us going down the slope with such devastating consequences.

We do know that the smallest act can have great repercussions for good and ill. That can be scary, but it can also be comforting because it means we don't have to wait for some world-shattering event to begin our recovery. The way to learn to walk is to take the First Step. And if we have been wounded, then we must learn to walk again, even if it means limping.

So let's start now. Let's light the spark that can change our world.

Today I'm ready to take the First Step toward a new life full of promise and hope.

PW

We shall not cease from exploration,
And the end of all our exploring
will be to arrive from where we started
And know the place for the first time.
— *T. S. Eliot*

What does a sex addict look like? How does a sex addict act? Newcomers often say how relieved they are to find that a sex addict isn't different from anyone else. In fact, walking into a meeting full of fear and shame and finding a fellowship of warm, honest, joyful people is often the first glimmer of hope for the addict who is still suffering.

We have a disease; it's called sex addiction. We're not to blame because we're addicts. We need never live in shame, no matter what we did in the past.

My recovery is restoring my dignity and self-esteem, One Day at a Time. I can give myself a lot of credit for having the courage to face my addiction.

SK

February

Do what you can, with what you have, where you are.

— *Theodore Roosevelt*

How often we wish we were someone else, living anywhere but here. We fantasize ourselves away from our centers into dreamy worlds of power, gratification, and ease. Frequently, our fantasies take a sexual turn and overpower us with images of control over others and easy self-gratification. We slide into a timeless world of selfish pleasure where real people cease to exist.

We all need to dream and daydream. But let's concentrate on living and enriching the here and now, rather than escaping into a passive world where people are mere objects to be manipulated. We now know the difference between sick and healthy relationships. This hard won knowledge can become healing wisdom as we strive toward a more fulfilling life.

I am learning to be attentive to the reality of the present moment and I live it as fully as I can.

PW

God, grant me the serenity
To accept the things I cannot change,
The courage to change the things I can,
And the wisdom to know the difference.
— *The Serenity Prayer*

"I'm in my addiction, and I don't know how to get out." To be that honest with ourselves, our sponsor, or our group is to start to find a way back. It's crucial to my recovery to know what my sex addiction is, how it acts, and how I feel when I'm in it. No one can put that awareness inside me but me.

To be in the addiction is painful, but we know that taking First Things First helps. Admitting that I'm power-less, calling someone, going to a meeting, and being gentle with myself are each important parts of my re-covery. Whatever works. Above all, I thank my Higher Power for the honesty and humility to admit that I'm struggling. It's all right to struggle; it's dangerous to stay in my addiction.

I am understanding that admitting when I struggle makes me strong. I know that the support I need to help me through my struggle is there if I ask for it.

SK

If a thing's worth doing, it's worth doing badly.
— *G. K. Chesterton*

It helps, sometimes, to turn a proverb upside down to see what happens. Many of us are brought up to believe that we have to perform, excel, finish first, get on the team, do a good job, see it through, get it done on time, say it right, get ahead, and on and on, better and better as we go. Why? Because that's the way Dad did it and Grandma did it and that's just the way it's supposed to be.

And then, inevitably, we'd fail or fall. So we'd turn back on ourselves in shame, beat ourselves up, run to drugs or addictive sex. If we were failures in public, then we'd make our own private world where failure didn't exist. In this little world fantasy ruled, and in fantasy there are only successes; everybody always scores. We once acted out our fantasies in secret or with anonymous partners who wouldn't tell anyone about our failures.

But it doesn't have to be so. We can break the spell, stop beating on ourselves, and get away from Father's angry voice or Mother's disappointed look. We can do things at our own speed, in our own way, one day at a time, just for the joy of doing them.

I'm fed up with perfectionism; I can enjoy my own abilities.

PW

Grief may be joy misunderstood;
Only the Good discerns the good.
— *Elizabeth Barrett Browning*

It may seem strange to grieve for the loss of our addiction, but there is indeed mourning that needs to take place as we recover. There is so much to let go of as we discover and admit the toll sex addiction has taken on our life. Letting go includes feeling this loss.

The challenge is to grieve without judging ourselves or our feelings. Maybe our addiction helped us cope with life when we didn't have healthy coping skills. Maybe it helped cover up feelings or events that were too painful to face. Maybe living as a practicing addict was truly the best we could do with our life at the time.

The tragedy was that as we sank deeper into addiction, it began to control us. It became our Higher Power, our lover, our job, our friend. That's why it's important to grieve not only for the loss of the addiction, no matter how unhealthy it was, but for the loss of ourselves and the things we missed out on in life because of our addiction. Grief, honestly felt and expressed, is a healing experience.

If I am grieving today, I give myself permission to do so. I need not be accountable to anyone else for how I feel, but I'll simply take care of myself with gentleness and compassion.

SK

*Success, recognition, and conformity are the
bywords of the modern world where everyone
seems to crave the anesthetizing security of
being identified with the majority.*
— *Martin Luther King*

When we were young, no doubt we sometimes felt
from our peers the pressure to conform. Perhaps we
were persuaded to try dope, to look at pornography,
to scorn the opposite sex, to laugh at those with more
conventional sexual attitudes — in a word, to be one
of the group. We felt different, unique, but we allowed
ourselves to be forced into a mold. Perhaps we were
lonely and we felt we needed the approval of our peers.
We didn't realize the cost to ourselves. But many of us
paid a price.

In recovery we need to reestablish our independence
and find out truly who we are. We will want to go back
to recover the lost child who went astray. At the same
time, we choose now to be part of a new community
of men and women working together to preserve their
independence. We can join this community freely and
still preserve our own identity as women and men.

---

*I am going to choose my own values and live my life
accordingly.*

PW

Understanding is the key to right principles and attitudes, and right action is the key to good living.
— Twelve Steps and Twelve Traditions

It can be easy to think of the Twelve Steps as an instructional guide, a manual for the recovering person: take Step One; then, Step Two; after that, Step Three — et cetera. They're not that at all. They're something we work on and experience our whole lives, One Day at a Time. We don't walk them once in a straight line.

The Twelve Steps are more like points on a circle; after we've taken the First Step, any one of them can be a beginning point, according to our needs. The fact that the Twelve Steps are a lifestyle, and that we are living them, forms the bond between us and other members of our group, whether we're a newcomer or an old-timer.

Rather than trying so hard to figure out the Steps and wondering if we're doing them right, we can listen to our hearts, and be grateful that there are Twelve Steps to guide us.

All the wisdom I need to change is found within the Steps, the fellowship, and myself with the help of my Higher Power.

SK

I love acting. It is so much more real than life.
— *Oscar Wilde*

Many of us sex addicts have gotten used to playing a part. We may hesitate to reveal our inmost selves because we are ashamed of who we really are. We can go through life with our true selves hidden by the masks of our false selves. Our illness has compelled us to be false, and we may have even taken pleasure in playacting. It may have made us feel good at times to know we're deceiving everyone around us, including our friends and loved ones. There were times when we fell in love with our own cleverness.

Sooner or later we became tired of being someone else. Our lovers, our children, and our friends became confused and hurt by our games and our inconstancy. They long to know us as we really are. As we gain the courage to get to know and love ourselves, we can drop our masks and let ourselves be seen and known and loved by others. Our lives, and theirs, will be richer.

I can be myself in public and private — especially with those I love.

PW

For so must it be, and help me to do my part.
— A Tibetan master

It's been said that God exists only in the present. That means we must live in the present if we are to find God. In God's eyes, we are worthy and lovable as we are, today. God never rejects part of creation.

Can we accept that our Higher Power loved us even when we were acting out? Can we accept that God loves us if we're struggling or even slipping today? If this happens, we can pick ourselves up and make the choice to go to a meeting, call a friend or a sponsor, or pray to our Higher Power.

The power of the present makes it possible for God to love us unconditionally because God doesn't expect us to be perfect, just willing to do our best. Only in the present do we have the power to choose our attitudes and actions, and it is this freedom that links us to God's power.

My Higher Power loves me because I'm human, not despite it.

SK

*Good people are good because they've come
to wisdom through failure.*
— *William Saroyan*

In our addiction we tend to think of other people as better than ourselves. We are quick to admire, to idealize. We are convinced that good people are good because they are born that way. And we, of course, are rotten.

But goodness comes through experience, and experience includes setbacks and even disasters. It's not so much what happens to us as the way we cope that makes the difference. What might be considered as failure can bring us to a deeper understanding of ourselves and other people.

Wisdom cannot be taught or transmitted; it comes directly from our personal experience in the world. And there we learn that goodness is a value extracted from the ordeals and adventures along our particular path. We can be quietly proud of our goodness.

I believe in my goodness and value as a member of the human family.

PW

*Love consists in this, that two solitudes protect
and touch and greet each other.*

— *Rilke*

A long-time member of the program talks about her
marriage: "My husband waited for me through seven
years of my acting out sexually until I finally got into
recovery. Then I waited three years for him to start dealing with his codependency.

"It's a mystery of the heart why we love each other.
Despite all the poor choices I'd made about men, I finally
married someone who has the gentleness, honesty, and
caring I need. I try not to analyze why we waited for
each other or how we stayed married all those years.
I just accept it, and now our relationship is the strongest
and best it has ever been."

Whether we're a recovering female or male sex addict, the hope in her story is ours to claim. If we want
and are waiting for a healthy relationship, we can believe
it will come when the time is right.

---

*I can work today to develop the qualities that will make
me a loving partner.*

SK

*The heart has reasons which reason does
not know.*

— *Pascal*

In a scientific age we rely on reason for explanation
of the world and our conduct. If our minds tell us
something is unreasonable, we tend not to do it. Our
heads rule our hearts.

But our hearts have voices, too, and they deserve
to be heard. Emotion is not just a force; it is also a
language whose words are often more powerful and
effective than those of the mind's language. Our hearts
can tell us about caring and affection and helping and
loving and being in touch.

In our addiction, we stopped listening to our hearts.
Our hearts themselves almost stopped. Recovery sets
the heart beating again in hope and love.

*I am coming to trust in the language of my heart — the
language of loving.*

PW

Feeling is the inner life; expression is the outer life.

— *Alexander Lowen*

There's a connection between our ability to feel, our ability to express our feelings, and our ability to let go. There are probably many painful emotions we learned to suppress when we were young, particularly anger or sadness. Other emotions might be difficult to feel because they're connected to past pain, especially about childhood sexual abuse or acting out in our addiction.

Yet there's no letting go, no moving on, until we stop trying to avoid feelings such as sorrow, anger, rage, or despair. One way to begin working through difficult feelings is to reach out to people with a phone call or by attending a meeting. Other ways are to write, have a good cry, plan a healing ritual, such as a couple days alone thinking. We can also remember to turn to our Higher Power for the spiritual help we need.

The release within that comes from expressing our feelings will help ease the pain. We can't let go of the past all at once, but we can let go of a little piece today.

If I'm hurting today, I can reach out for the healing of the program. I will give myself the same compassion I would give another person who is suffering.

SK

*There is plenty of courage among us in the
abstract but not in the concrete.*
— *Helen Keller*

In our minds we are often the bravest people in the
world and we daily do great deeds there. Usually it is
the grand gesture that captures our fancy and wins us
great renown — in our imagination. And we wait for
the day when we can prove our courage to the world.

In the meantime, what about our addiction? Do we
continue to sit alone wrapped up in our sexual fantasies? Do we go on acting out at the expense of others?
Do we flee intimacy and hide from honesty? Are we
out of control?

Let's take a hard look at the things we *can* change in
our sexuality. We may not yet understand why we act
as we do, but we know what we want to change. We
want to integrate our sexuality into the rest of our lives
and not have it split off and ruining us. That is something where courage is needed — and needed every day.

*I want to focus in on my addiction and apply courage to
the daily steps of my recovery.*

PW

Every forward step we take we leave some phantom of ourselves behind.
— *John Spalding*

A recovering person once remarked that every day when he woke up, he said, "Okay, God, surprise me." Although each day brings new challenges, there is one thing it won't bring — perfection. Today, we can expect a mixed bag of experiences with a wide range of emotions to match.

If we're feeling discouraged or negative about our life, one way to cultivate an attitude of gratitude is to look back and see how far we've come. Remember, we seek progress, not perfection. There is always something to be grateful for, including the ability to find something to be grateful for.

When life is so bad that I want to cry, I'll try laughing instead.

SK

To live a life half dead, a living death.
— *John Milton*

Sex addiction, like any other addiction, may have given us, for a moment, the illusion of being really alive. Then, after acting out, we plunged back into passivity. Our fantasies and our acting out can make us high, and that's why our addiction is so hard to view objectively and why it is so hard to begin recovery. But we know that while in our addiction we are only half alive, locked away in the closet of our fantasies and obsessive thinking. And half alive means half dead.

To go through life half dead is to deny the most precious gift we have — the possibility of living life joyfully and abundantly. We are capable of so many things, in our work, at rest, with our friends and loved ones, at play. We can dance, cry, laugh, sing, paint, ski, travel, rest, cook, help others, walk, talk. . .there are a thousand ways to spend an hour, a day, a life.

Much of this glory would be lost if we chose to remain closed off from life in our addiction. When we take the First Step on the path of recovery, we enrich our lives and the lives of those around us.

Each day I can come back to life and live more fully and joyfully.

PW

You can't drive straight on a twisting lane.
— *Russian proverb*

What did it take to bring us to the point where we were willing to admit our powerlessness and unmanageability over our addiction to sex? Most of us did not reach this point until we faced some horrible consequences not once, but over and over.

Even in recovery, our denial can be strong. If we approach our addiction only intellectually, without acknowledging our feelings, our chances for staying in denial are much greater. We can't rewrite the story of our life, and we can't wipe out the painful memories. Whatever we've done is done, and when we face up to that reality honestly, we can face up to powerlessness. We can reach out and ask for help, and we can start to help ourselves.

Admitting my powerlessness over my addiction offers me a way back from my addiction. It is an invitation to accept myself as I am and to go on from there.

SK

The handwriting on the wall may be a forgery.
— *Ralph Hodgson*

Too often we addicts are superstitious and interpret signs in negative or hostile ways. Because we don't believe in ourselves, we tend to think that fate is against us.

But life isn't for us or against us. If we are attentive we will see many signs of promise during each day. Signs of promise, signs of goodness, signs of beauty. And if we trust ourselves and our Higher Power, we will know how to interpret the world and use it to do good.

Sometimes we may be unsure of our next step or even our general direction. If we are patient and alert to the world around us, we will pick up hints and clues that will help us on our way — a friend's telephone call, a warm hug, a chance encounter, a job offer, a word of advice from a loved one. When we are ready, we'll know how to respond and what to do.

One thing we are learning to be sure of: in this world of signs, we are not alone.

I don't want to believe in a hostile fate. The world is good and I am finding my way in it by being patient and learning to read the signs.

PW

What is the deepest loss you have suffered?
If drinking is bitter, change yourself to wine. . . .
And if the earthly no longer knows your name,
whisper to the silent earth: I'm flowing.
To the flashing water say: I am.

— *Rilke*

It's not that we want God to change everything about us or remake us to perfection. (OK, maybe we do.) It's not that we wish we were other than who we are; some days we even like who we are. It's more that we want to have faith in ourselves, a deep-down, constant faith that steadies us. We want to have roots deep in the earth, not fragile roots of glass.

Strong and deep roots are made of self-esteem, hope, love, willingness, humility, and faith. Our longing to be grounded in life may take the form of wishing we were not addicted to sex, but that's a cover-up for the deeper things we truly want.

Recovery reorganizes our personalities, indeed our very souls, around new, spiritual principles. We remain sex addicts and always will be, yet that doesn't prevent us from possessing faith in ourselves and the courage to keep growing.

I am a vessel containing life. I am a vessel that has been shattered and mended. I will endure.

SK

If they try to rush me, I always say, "I've only got one other speed — and it's slower."
— Glenn Ford

We tend to feel ourselves under pressure to perform, to produce, to excel. But pressure makes us feel rushed, and we become careless with ourselves and with others. We miss seeing and enjoying the small, simple things in life. We get things and people out of focus.

Pressure can come from inside too — from our shame and sense of unworthiness. Then we find it difficult to look the world in the eye because of our secretive sexual lives. We may feel we have to keep moving in order to prevent ourselves from assessing the true nature of our illness and the harm it did to ourselves and others.

But now we know we can slow down and take each day, each hour and minute as it comes. By slowing down, we learn to see the world more clearly and enjoy the company of others. We do have time to get to know ourselves and reach out to others. The reward is a deeper, quieter, lovelier life.

Time is not an enemy to be conquered, but part of the rhythm of life. Each day I try to slow down and live.

PW

I don't want the cheese, I just want to get out of the trap.

— *Spanish proverb*

Sex addiction has two sides: one side is acting out; the other is trying to control our acting out in order to control our addiction. When we were acting out, we tried to control ourselves through willpower and intellect. Now we have much healthier ways to live, ways that include the knowledge that there is no way to control an addiction. The only choice is to let go of it.

We get all the time we need to define what abstinence is for us. There may be days in recovery when all we can do is white-knuckle it in order to keep from acting out. Our abstinence may not be what we wish it were, but as long as we're taking care of ourselves and not acting out, we're abstinent. Later, our abstinence will grow and deepen to include reclaiming our sexuality in new, nonaddictive ways. One thing we do know: However we define our abstinence, without it there is no recovery.

I know I can't control my addiction, but I can let go of it with my Higher Power's help. I define my abstinence with this in mind. I am willing to stay abstinent today.

SK

What loneliness is more lonely than distrust?
— *George Eliot*

Part of our isolation as sex addicts comes from our lack of trust. When we were children, many of us went to adults with openness and confidence and were turned away, abandoned, or abused. We shrank away from contact because touch may have been associated with seduction or harm. We retreated into the deep isolation of despair.

How can we move outward again? When we come to our groups, we have the opportunity to meet with others one-on-one, or in smaller groups, as well as in larger groups. We can find a sponsor, talk on the telephone, and meet group members for breakfast. Gradually we come into contact with people who do not hurt us, abandon us, or abuse us.

An essential part of our recovery is regaining confidence in other people, and this takes time. But we have time. And we have the place and the people. Our Twelve Step group is the basis for a new, trusting relationship with the world.

I know it takes time to break out of isolation and to learn to trust people, but I know it can be done — and I can do it.

PW

God delays, but doesn't forget.
                     — Spanish proverb

It's frustrating to get sick, lose a job, or encounter financial setbacks. We suddenly feel curtailed, with the rhythm of our lives changed in a way we never anticipated. But our Higher Power slows us down for a reason.

There can be gifts in adversity. They can provide us with time alone, time to think. Being alone gives us the chance to find ourselves in a new way. We may be surprised to find inner resources we didn't know we had. A period of waiting through adversity can also turn us to God when the solace we need is beyond the capacity of people to give.

It's challenging to be able to do nothing when the world tells us that we must always take action. When action isn't possible, accepting the circumstances of our lives enables us to experience the value of being, rather than doing.

When some part of my life is beyond my control, I can be patient and simply wait. Inaction is not necessarily inactivity.

SK

In the difficult are the friendly forces, the hands that work on us.

— *Rilke*

Too often we imagine life as a magic carpet taking us wherever we wish to go. Perhaps we are watching television and an advertisement hooks into our fantasy and convinces us that the world is at our beck and call. We are omnipotent again as we were in infancy — "Your Majesty the Baby."

But what would such a magical life yield in terms of change and growth? Why would we bother to strive if we could have everything we crave? We would be the same at fifty as we were at thirty and fifteen and five months — "Your Majesty the Baby."

We need change and most of us welcome it, even if change means growing pains. With the guidance of our Higher Power we can strive toward goodness. We are not omnipotent, but we are not alone. We are part of a human community, and we can be in touch with a Power beyond ourselves. That is the real miracle.

I'm not afraid of what is difficult, provided it helps me grow.

PW

Love your self's self where it lives.
— *Anne Sexton*

How often have we wished we were someone else, anyone else, rather than who we are? If we're intense, have we longed to be calmer? If we're introverted, have we dreamed of being extroverted? And, of course, being a sex addict, have we wished we were "normal"?

The truth is that there is no such thing as "normal." Each of us is special; we have the potential within to realize our unique destiny. The infinite growth of which we're capable comes from qualities we now possess. We can change ourselves, but we can never put within us what simply isn't there. To try to do so is perfectionistic and will focus our energy outside ourselves, which can trigger our addiction.

Instead, we can learn to be directed by what is inside of us. We can appreciate and love ourselves as we are and choose people in our life who do the same.

The more I appreciate the mystery of who I am, the less I'll wish I were someone else.

SK

*Sin has many tools, but a lie is the handle that
fits them all.*

— *Oliver Wendell Holmes, Jr.*

If we are addicted to sex, chances are that our lives
are built on lying. We all have many shortcomings, but
when we are addicted, lying rules supreme. We are so
ashamed of our behavior that we flee the truth and, even
in the smallest things, automatically turn to a lie.

Lying is an offense against life and those we love. Why
can't we look our beloved in the eye? Why do we turn
away from our children and deceive them in our shame?

Our program insists on rigorous honesty from the
very beginning. We must be honest, with ourselves and
with our fellow sufferers. In the community of our
recovery group, as we speak the truth fearlessly and
openly, we gradually come to terms with ourselves and
learn to be there for others.

Lying cuts us off from others; the truth binds us
together.

---

*I am tired of lying when I look into the eyes of those who
trust me. I know I can learn to be honest and come to trust
in myself and in the truth.*

PW

*Love must be learned, and learned again and
again; there is no end to it. Hate needs no in-
struction, but only waits to be provoked.*
— *Katherine Anne Porter*

We often enter into our relationships believing there
is one perfect way to act, and if we can only find that
way, we'll be successful, accepted. But there is no such
thing as "one best way" to be with another person. The
wonder of any relationship is that it involves two imperfect people.

Believing that perfection will ensure love is addictive
thinking. Love is a gift that must be given freely; there
is nothing we can do to control someone else's choice
to love us or not love us. All we can do is our part by
learning each day to love as best we can. It may be
difficult to find within ourselves such qualities as emotional maturity, separateness, honesty, forgiveness,
patience, and self-respect. But those are the very qualities we must cultivate to love someone else.

It can be frightening to trust another person enough
to take risks and let go of the outcome. But love is a
risk that's worth it.

---

*I am learning that I don't need to be perfect to be accepted
and loved by others. I'm also learning that I don't need to
expect perfection from others to love and accept them.*

SK

When I grow up I want to be a little boy.
— *Joseph Heller*

As children, our sexuality may have been something we feared or ignored, abused or repressed. We may not have felt at home with our sexual feelings, as if they didn't belong to us. Perhaps they were stolen from us by a person who abused us sexually.

These feelings may have made us not want to be children as they prevented us from really enjoying our childhood. As such, we came to be ill at ease with the child within us, wanting to forget, reject, and abandon him or her all over again.

But the child in us all is a living, vital, creative part of us that we need to be in touch with to feel whole again. We might want to carry a photograph of ourselves as a child so that we may be reminded of who we were and who in some ways we still are. That child needs us, and we need that child to continue to play and create and love.

I want to bring the child alive in me and let it grow throughout my life.

PW

*A spirituality that is divorced from the body
becomes an abstraction, just as a body denied
its spirituality becomes an object.*
— Alexander Lowen

When we were acting out, we often treated other people as objects. We chose partners or relationships based on externals: Was she beautiful? Was he handsome? Was the person someone we'd want on our arm at a party? And, of course, the most important criterion: Could we possibly act out with this person?

We treated ourselves as objects too, caring more about how we looked or what people thought of us than what we thought of ourselves. We had no genuine sense of dignity because we were locked in a fantasy world, looking for the perfect sexual experience.

As we recover, we have realized we are not just a body, and our body is not an object. We are each a human being with feelings, needs, and a point of view. We deserve to treat ourselves and others with respect, remembering our common dignity as people.

I am seeing myself as a whole person, which helps me see other people that way too.

SK

Whenever one finds oneself inclined to bitterness, it is a sign of emotional failure.
— *Bertrand Russell*

We sometimes meet bitter and cynical people who may amuse us for a while. They seem so sure of themselves and so full of the experience of the world.

But when we get to know these people better, we realize that they are really frightened of feeling — and fearful of life. Their bitterness masks an inability to be in touch with themselves and others.

Sex addiction made us bitter, since it blocked our real feelings with the mechanical actions of our obsessions. We felt shameful and incurable, and our attitudes became arid and hostile. Real feelings dried up, and we turned away in fear from love and life.

Our recovery helps us release our emotions and respond honestly and directly to others and the world around us. Each day we expand our emotional range because we are no longer afraid.

I know that bitterness and cynicism are insults to life; I want to continue to reach out to the world with true feeling.

PW

March

The words "I am. . ." are potent words; be careful what you hitch them to. The thing you're claiming has a way of reaching back and claiming you.

— *A. L. Kitselman*

Today is our chance to leave the past behind and live in the present. It doesn't matter what we did as a practicing sex addict. If we're abstinent today, if we're working our program today, if we're doing the best we can today, that's all that counts.

It's easy to live in the shame and negativity of the past without even realizing it. But those days are over — we don't live that life anymore. We can forgive ourselves or someone else today and let our changed life be our amend for the past.

Forgiveness, gratitude, intimacy, gentleness, honesty: these are the gifts we give to ourselves and others when we live in the present.

How do I feel right now? Do I feel serene or is there something bothering me? Being honest about what's going on with me is a good way to live in the present.

SK

The mass of men lead lives of quiet desperation.
— Henry David Thoreau

As we became more deeply immersed in our addiction, we were more desperate in our search for relief and in our flight from responsibility. Cruising, videos, pornographic images, anonymous encounters — all are acts of despondency and despair, without love and without hope.

In recovery, we need to be utterly fearless in our self-examination and balanced in the inventory we take of ourselves. We can share the exact nature of our wrongs and our progress in recovery with another human being and with our Higher Power. And we can be specific about our addiction and at the same time talk about our strong points. The path to recovery leads through an honest look at our character defects and the reconsideration of our beliefs and values.

Honesty about ourselves and admission of our shortcomings to others lead to a sense of reconnecting with the truth of ourselves and with the human community where real, vital people live and love.

All is well when I greet myself and others as members of the human community.

PW

Life delights in life.
— William Blake

How do we connect with other people? Do we rely on conflict, suffering, manipulation, gossip, one-upmanship? Do we create relationships that can be controlled safely, and then call that "reality"?

Real connection requires two people, both wanting to be in the relationship, to approach each other as equals. A good relationship brings us happiness, growth, and a satisfying feeling of closeness. We are able to be ourselves, without adjusting our beliefs or behavior to please the other person or to maintain the relationship. The moment we abandon our equality, we have a power struggle, not a relationship.

When we acted out, the only connection we made was between us and the addictive hunger, an appetite that was never filled. In recovery, we can connect with other people, giving and receiving, and finding the joy that comes with true connection.

There is a triangle in my relationships: myself, the other person, and my Higher Power. I can trust the connection I feel, giving what I can without worrying about what I may receive in return.

SK

All the fame I look for in life is to have lived it quietly.

— *Montaigne*

The desire for fame can often be distracting. We can be so busy striving to be recognized that we lose sight of ourselves. What comes to mind is what other people think of us; we defer to their opinion, and neglect our own intimate view of ourselves.

Being well-thought-of is fine and good. . .as long as we think well of ourselves. We need to tend our own garden and love what grows therein. Having it admired by the neighbors is nice but not always necessary.

A quiet life brings us into touch with ourselves. We come to realize how much we are worth in our own eyes. With this confidence in ourselves, we can reach out and love — not because we are empty and needy, but because we believe in our own uniqueness and value.

I resolve to seek quietness and the love that springs from self-knowledge.

PW

What I wanted
Was to be myself again.
— Sandra Hochman

When we lose faith in our feelings, we lose faith in ourselves and become outer-directed. We look to the world to tell us what to do, and how to feel. We seek approval and love from others so we can prove to ourselves that we're worthy. Paradoxically, to be outer-directed is to be self-absorbed. Because we feel so unsure of who we are, we cannot let go and be spontaneous, real.

The task in recovery is to reclaim ourselves by becoming inner-directed. This means looking within for the direction we need. When we're just learning to trust our feelings, this can be truly agonizing. It means trusting the reality of our needs and our right to express them. Only then can we find the faith in ourselves and in life that we have lacked.

To become inner-directed takes self-acceptance and self-love. It also takes time. But there is no real peace otherwise, for it is the only way to find ourselves.

I can be true to my own feelings. I am my own best teacher because I know what I truly need.

SK

*Such is the human race. Often it does seem
such a pity that Noah... didn't miss the boat.*
— *Mark Twain*

Was it a pity? Would it have been better if humanity
had disappeared in the Flood? Perhaps if we are in the
depths of our addiction we may be tempted to agree
— people are rotten, sex is wretched, we're no good,
life is vile. On the days we dwell in the misery of our
shame, the world does indeed seem a dark and gloomy
dungeon.

This is the misery of sex addiction: it takes the heart
and guts out of our lives and turns the world into a place
of shadows and despair. Then, everything we do is
marked and marred by our feelings of unworthiness
and melancholy.

But we know there is a way out. We must open up
to others in recovery and speak our pain and our sorrow. We can be sure that they will listen to us because
they have been there before; and now they are here,
for us. When our addiction seems like a flood that God
has sent into our lives, our program can be our Ship
of Hope. As we join our new companions, our First Step
will be the beginning of a new life.

*When I rise above my addiction I see the world in a new
light.*

It is the creative potential itself in human beings
that is the image of God.

— Mary Daly

Within each of us is a creative person. Getting comfortable with our creativity often means letting go of tight, rigid thinking so the spontaneous, artistic side of ourselves can emerge.

Whether or not we think of ourselves as artistic, we are. To be artistic is to create, an instinct we all possess. Each day in recovery we find the courage to create ourselves anew. One way to encourage our creativity is to find an outlet for it. It may be playing the piano, embroidering, gardening, or refinishing furniture. Most anything that lets us create something outside ourselves can be good.

The joy of working with our body, spirit, mind, and feelings is truly a joyful experience with an amazing reward at the end: we find we have created something new, and in it, we can see ourselves.

I am letting go of the rigid ways of thinking that prevent my creativity from emerging. My creativity is more important to me than rigid ways of thinking.

SK

If you cannot get rid of the family skeleton, you may as well make it dance.
— *George Bernard Shaw*

Many sex addicts come from families with secrets and hidden shame. Sometimes for generations there has been no open discussion of feelings, no direct and honest exchanges among family members. A system of unspoken messages and hidden guilt surrounds the children in these families. They become more and more alone.

In our solitude we used to see ourselves as bad people because we picked up the message that our sexuality was somehow wrong and shameful. Our desire was turned back to be hidden, and we were always at war with ourselves. We became a battlefield for a civil war that we always lost.

We get out of this unhealthy isolation when we learn to talk about our backgrounds and our places within our family system. If there are skeletons, we rattle them a little and shake them up. We even learn to laugh at the crazy world of shame and repression that kept us away from life. In talking and laughing we begin to break free.

I want to be free of the guilt and shame that keep me bound to an addictive cycle.

PW

*I look in the mirror through the eyes of the child
that was me.*

— *Judy Collins*

It's been said that the primary task of a parent is to awaken the spirit of the child. Many of us were raised by parents who did anything but that. Indeed, their actions may have broken our spirits.

As parents ourselves, we have another chance. We have a child within us who remembers pain that a child should never have to feel. And we have a child inside who remembers innocence and joy. The view of the joyful, innocent child is the gift we can give our children. We can give them the gentleness, respect, and empathy they deserve. We do not live through our children; they are separate people with lives of their own. But we can awaken their spirits by showing them the unconditional love that we feel for them and that they long to receive from us.

When I treat myself well, I'm able to treat my children well. I am learning to give myself and my children the care and understanding needed to nurture our spirits.

SK

Within our dreams and aspirations we find our opportunities.

— Sue Atchley Ebaugh

Many great creative people, such as Einstein, have made important discoveries while daydreaming. We also can tap into the energy that comes from random associations and the unconscious. Through this, a new vision becomes possible.

Perhaps when we were at school we were told to be alert and not to dream our lives away. Parents, too, may have discouraged our imaginative lives. Our culture tends to reward the rational and the pragmatic and to consider the dreamer of marginal importance.

But let's not lose our power to dream. Our dreams can be much more than sexual fantasies born of our addiction. Our deepest wishes and hopes will often come to the surface when we are drowsing or simply letting the mind roam through life's possibilities. Many times we stumble on the truth in our dreams. We need the energy and the vision that come with dreaming.

I welcome the gift of ideas that come to me while giving my imagination free play.

PW

True hope is swift, and flies with
swallows wings
      — *William Shakespeare*

When we read the words "restore us to sanity" in Step Two, we can believe absolutely that somewhere within us, we are sane. Restoration means returning to us what we already possess — wholeness. Through this Step we find the beginnings of reconciliation; we are reconciled with ourselves and our Higher Power, and we have the hope of being reconciled with other people.

Working this Step takes patience because it is a process, sometimes a long one. Coming to believe doesn't mean embracing a body of intellectual beliefs; it means beginning to find faith, which is entirely different from intellectual belief. Before we can have faith, we must have hope. This Step provides that.

Like a child, I take one Step at a time. I believe that today my life is being restored to me.

SK

I know well what I am fleeing from but not what I am in search of.

— *Montaigne*

Many of us are aware that we no longer wish to go on being the person who is addicted to sex, often seeming to act independently of our wills and values. We flee that person who we know is destructive and self-absorbed. We are turning against that automaton.

We may not know exactly what we desire all the time, or who we wish to be. In any case, we've learned there will not ever be a fixed and final moment that provides the answer to our search. What matters is that we are moving away from destructive habits and disheartening patterns. We are learning to listen to others and to our own inner voices. We are on the move.

We do not have to have a rigid plan to continue along the path of recovery and the joy of a new life.

In turning away from my old habits, I see the amazing possibilities of a new life to be lived.

PW

In every person, even in such that appear most reckless, there is an inherent desire to attain balance.

— *Jakob Wasserman*

In contrast to compulsivity is inactivity. Since many of us tend toward compulsivity, do we sometimes find ourselves going to the other extreme and not doing anything? Not doing anything is one way to try to control our addiction. It can be difficult to get going once we no longer use sex as our energizer. It can be just as difficult to slow down if we substitute mindless activity for sex in order to dull our feelings.

What we need is the faith that life is safe, and that we are safe within it. We also need the energy that comes from a Power greater than ourselves. There is a healthy balance that is neither the activity of compulsion nor the inactivity of fear and control. When we are moving to our own internal rhythm, we feel a serenity that brings the pleasure of the present into focus and lets us enjoy it.

What do I need today? If I must get going, I can act as if. If I want to slow down, I can let myself stop and take a break.

SK

One deceit needs many others, and so the whole house is built in the air and must soon come crashing down.

— *Baltasar Gracián.*

If we are honest about our addiction, we know how it can drive us into secrecy. At first came the little lie — about missing an appointment or coming home late. Then the lie to cover the lie, and then the lies to try to escape from the web of lies that entangled us within our deceit. We couldn't look our loved one in the eye, we couldn't risk the truth, and so we lied again and again. Finally the sad day came when we grew comfortable in our little isolated world of fantasy and deception.

Our life became a house of cards, a pack of lies. We couldn't make an honest, open move for fear of bringing the whole thing tumbling down around our ears. And usually we were not the only ones to get hurt; our spouses, lovers, children, friends, and colleagues suffered too.

We have begun to change all this, but it takes time. We need to continue to take inventory and be fearless and honest with ourselves. Each time we are honest, the lies lose their power, and finally truth comes through.

I'm tired of the web of lies I've spun around my addiction. I want to break through into honesty and truth.

To gain that which is worth having, it may be
necessary to lose everything else.
— Bernadette Devlin

It is a humbling experience to admit there is a Power greater than ourselves. We felt powerful as a sex addict, especially when we were acting out. But that power was an illusion; we used it to hide the truth. We truly believed that our addiction was all-powerful. It was the force we counted on and protected.

What an undertaking then to admit our powerlessness and to acknowledge our need for a Power greater than ourselves. Our life can feel like a battleground, with our addiction pulling us one way and our recovery urging us another. And where is God during this struggle? Our Higher Power, unlike our addiction, does not force us to do anything, but waits until we choose. We do not have to take action any particular way; we will decide to turn our life over to the care of our Higher Power as we're ready. We need only sense a spiritual presence ready to help us when we are ready to accept our powerlessness.

Step Two is a way for me to start to know my own spirituality.
Can I accept this gift from my Higher Power?

SK

It is not our exalted feelings, it is our senti-
ments that build the necessary home.
— *Elizabeth Bowen*

When we felt high because of our addiction, we let
out our emotions in extravagant, exalted ways, and we
thought we were getting in touch with our feelings.
But, in fact, we were only getting in touch with our high;
our real feelings were forgotten and unused. And after
awhile we discounted our real feelings altogether, in favor
of our artificial emoting.

Part of our healing process is the rediscovery of deep
reservoirs of feeling that have always been part of our
inheritance but that have become dammed up and
thwarted by our addiction. We have been operating on
false sentiments and affections. Our disease has turned
us away from our true selves.

When we say, in the Second Step, that we can be restored to sanity, we are talking about our true feelings,
among other things. As a result of our program, we will
find that once again we can laugh and cry and express
sorrow and anger and joy. The dam has burst; we are
released from the killing power of our addiction.

I am learning to distinguish between the false exaltation
that comes from my addiction and true feelings that come
directly from my heart.

PW

*You cannot step twice into the same river, for
other waters are continually flowing on.*
— Heraclitus

How we see ourselves and the words we use to describe ourselves are important. If we label ourselves "a sex addict," will we feel and act like a sex addict? Although it can be a great relief to find a name for our addiction, we want to be careful not to use those words against ourselves.

The words "sex addict" are only words. The reality we bring to them is our own. The words may be emotionally charged for us and other people, but in the end they only describe a part of who we are. They don't describe us entirely.

Every moment of recovery is a transition between the old us and the new us. When we want to move away from an image of ourselves as addicts and see ourselves as whole people, we can do that. To do so does not mean we deny the reality of our addiction; it means we see a more complete picture of who we are.

I can be a grateful addict today, knowing it was my addiction that brought me a new life.

SK

There are no elements so diverse that they can-
not be joined in the heart of an individual.
— Jean Giraudoux

We sometimes look too hard, perhaps, for unity and coherence. If we are uncertain, we get upset; if we are inconsistent, we are criticized. So we try to always be constant and predictable.

But we are made up from disparate genes and conflicting humors. We may always want to do good, but we all have slips. Our hearts say one thing, our heads another. We change our minds and stop and start. We get confused and battles flare up inside us.

That's called being human. Many forces converge on us, many thoughts arise, many emotions rage. It takes courage to accept our contradictions, our struggles, but we will be stronger if we do.

I recognize that I am often divided in myself. I accept that this is part of being human.

PW

All day, where the sunlight played on the
seashore, Life sat.
— *Olive Schreiner*

When we let ourselves, we look around and feel a
deep sense of respect for life and our part in it. The
land — its majesty and sustenance — children, pets, doing something we love: all of these nourish our spirit.

It's important to find the things that nurture our spirit
and do them, and it's important to keep widening the
possibilities for awakening our spirit. The excitement
that arises from a moment of connection is wonderful
to feel. Although the moment can be simple, something
we wouldn't have noticed in the past, we can now feel
its reality. The deepest part of us reaches out to something or someone else, and we are connected. Intimacy
with life renews life.

God, please help me today to say yes to the beauty, people
and experiences in my life.

SK

Whenever he thought about Vietnam, he felt terrible. And so, at last, he came to a fateful decision. He decided not to think about it.
— *Anonymous*

There are many things we may not like to think about, and often whole societies try to pretend that some things don't exist. The Victorians, publicly at least, tended to deny the force and attraction of sexuality, which led to many taboos.

The effects of these taboos are still felt by many of us. We may be unable to speak openly about sex, or even to think sanely about it in the privacy of our own minds. And if we don't get it straight in our thoughts, we can't feel at home with it or manage our lives.

Talking helps. We need a secure and loving environment in which to articulate our fears and our longings, our remorse and our aspirations. When we come to that place and meet others afflicted by sex addiction, we feel the beginning of a healing process that is the start of a new life.

I don't want to run away from unpleasant thoughts and realities. In facing the truth I can begin to be free.

PW

No is an affirmation of life just as yes is. Only falsehood is death. Lying to oneself is a defect of the spirit.

— Romain Rolland

Every day we pray for the willingness to make sane choices about our sexuality. In the morning, when we awaken, the way we feel gives us an idea of whether the day will be easy or difficult. If we're not feeling our strongest, we need to take special care of our abstinence that day.

That might mean a phone call, writing out how we plan to confront a difficult situation, writing affirmations to take with us, and thinking ahead to potential danger. Do we need to avoid a certain part of town, make a contract not to call an old lover, or stay away from certain music? If we're planning to go to a movie this evening, do we need to choose the movie with extra care? Persons, places, things, and events that can trigger our addiction are everywhere, and it's up to us to act before, not react after. Our abstinence is a gift to be cared for and strengthened, One Day at a Time.

There are days when maintaining abstinence is more difficult than other days. On these days I will take special care to ensure my abstinence.

SK

Forgiveness is the key to action and freedom.
— *Hannah Arendt*

Part of our recovery is the difficult quest for forgiveness. Our addiction caused us to do harmful things to ourselves and others. We were angry and rude and perhaps treacherous and hateful.

How can we find forgiveness? Can we ever find forgiveness for all our wrongs? Let's go slowly and start by looking at ourselves. We have been hard on ourselves and without mercy for our failings — but many of them come from the illness of our sex addiction. We were a battleground for self-hatred. We split ourselves into two persons: the one who acts out, and the one who condemns. Forgiveness brings those two warring selves back together again.

Now we are ready to make a list of those who have been harmed by us in our addiction. They will not always forget, nor will we. But we can reach out to them in love and humility. With these burdens of harm and hate removed, we are ready to move out into the active world of freedom.

I want to forgive myself for hurting myself and those I love.

PW

I tell you, the great divide is still with us, the awful split, the Us and Them....The polarization of the sexes continues because we lack the courage to face our likenesses and admit to our real need.

— Colette Dowling

We look into his face, and we see the Other. We look into her eyes, and we see the Difference Between Us. As recovering sex addicts, we have known the pain of disconnection from other people. Why, then, would we want to continue that disconnection by not having people of the other sex in our lives? No matter what our sexual boundaries may be, the gifts men and women receive from each other are many and invaluable.

A way to start is to have friends of the other sex. With friends we can be ourselves. We can make mistakes; we can share activities; we can talk. We can call on and support in each other the subtleties and strengths that are the very essence of masculinity and femininity. And we can do it because we are different sexes.

Is there someone of the other sex I'd like for a friend? I can take the risk by reaching out to him or to her.

SK

*Honesty is the first chapter of the book
of wisdom.*

— *Thomas Jefferson*

We have to find our own way to wisdom, and the road may sometimes seem long and hard. How do we start? How far do we have to go? How do we know when we are there?

Most of us find it helpful to travel the road with others, in a Twelve Step group. There we learn to be honest with ourselves and to trust our inner voice. After a time we are able to separate fact from fantasy and come to a mature perspective on our own conduct.

We need courage to be rigorously honest. It is so easy to gloss over yesterday's slip or forget that our behavior has hurt a loved one. We may wish to begin by listing our good and bad qualities. This helps us get a sense of proportion and provides the basis for an assessment of those actions that have harmed others and ourselves. Then we can decide about making amends to the people we have hurt. Going one step at a time takes away our fear that we can never do it, never get there. Honesty, like anything else, can be learned, with patience and love.

I want to learn honesty as a vital step on the path to wisdom and serenity.

PW

I have never, in all my life, been so odious as to regard myself as "superior" to any living being, human or animal.

— Edith Sitwell

Would we rather be more right than anyone else? The desire to be right, born of perfectionism, pride and fear, can trap us. We find ourselves making untenable choices: we'd rather be right — even if it means risking a friendship. We absolutely know we're correct — to the point of alienating our boss. Or we refuse to admit we're wrong — even if we hurt a loved one. We'd rather be right than be loved.

A rigid need to be right is really self-righteousness in disguise. What we sometimes call "standing up for our principles" is really inflexibility. It is a relief to let go of the search for the one right way to do things. Suddenly, we find ourselves noticing what we share with others instead of our differences. Listening with an open mind and lessening our stake in being right automatically brings us closer to other people; it takes down yet another barrier.

Noticing when I need to be right will help me become aware of my own self-righteousness. Not being right doesn't mean I'm weak.

SK

Earth's crammed with heaven
And every common bush afire with God.
　　　— Elizabeth Barrett Browning

We are taught that earth is here and heaven is "up there," and so we divide our world. There's a time and a place for everything — each in its own compartment. God's in His Heaven and all's right with the world!

But experience contradicts this simple view. As we grow and explore the world we can't make such clear distinctions anymore. We come to see that the world is a place where the divine may be present or absent, depending on our perception and even our mood. In the depths of our addiction we may find an emptiness and a darkness that deny the presence of any meaning at all.

In recovery, as we reach out, the world takes on a different color and feeling. As we gain confidence and dare to be happy, we find a new sense of power and love. And when joy comes to us, we share the poet's vision of a world in which many simple things are indeed "afire with God."

As I gain hope and faith, the world turns into a place of splendor and praise.

PW

Sorrow you can hold, however desolating, if nobody speaks to you. If they speak to you, you break down.

— Bede Jarrett

Who among us has not known the loneliness of this addiction: the shame, the despair, the feeling of utter abandonment by other people, and the terror of being out of control? When calling an old lover or finding ourselves in the wrong part of town, we feel fearful, separate, we think, "I'm not like other people; they don't do these things." This is the message of our addiction. It says to us, "You are an outcast. You need me because you're nothing without me. You're worthless."

As we recover, we discover that our addiction is a liar. We are not worthless, and we are not alone. We are a group of people recovering together, helping each other along.

And so, when you are in pain and unable to speak, I will be your voice. You will be my voice. I will be your heart. You will be my heart. We will hold each other up, and we, with the help of a Higher Power, will quite literally love each other into recovery.

God, I thank You for bringing me into recovery. Let me show You my gratitude by growing in my recovery.

SK

She lives on the reflections of herself in the eyes of others. She doesn't dare to be herself.
— Anaïs Nin

Do I know myself only in the image of what others make of me? Do I exist only in the gaze of others? What would happen if there was nobody to see me, to make me up? Would I simply disappear and cease to exist?

If we lack a sense of ourselves as people changing, on the move, in a process of growth, then it is easy to let ourselves become fixed, defined, static, lifeless. Other people will always be happy to do the work of defining us if we are unwilling to find out who we are ourselves.

Of course we need to be seen and noticed and valued by others — but not at the expense of ourselves. We must dare to be. We must take the risk of creating ourselves and get to know and like ourselves — this strange and wonderful creature.

I am going to dare to be myself and welcome change and growth.

PW

I never found the companion that was so companionable as solitude.
— Henry David Thoreau

There will be times when we find ourselves alone, despite our best efforts to reach out. That's often when we most need help, and it's usually when nobody is home or it's the middle of the night. The reality of being alone can lead to panic and to the belief we will be alone forever. But after the initial fear passes, we need to believe we can take care of ourselves. We have many more resources in us than we may realize.

If we ask ourselves what we really need, we'll find an answer. It may be a walk, doing the dishes, sitting down with our journal, or praying. It may even be finding the courage to experience our feelings all alone and let go of the outcome.

The voice that tells us we can't manage alone will have its say, but it can't run the show. Our inner voice, by which we know what's best for us, is doing that.

If I am unable to be with others, I will accept that and be with myself. I may just find I'm pretty nice to be with.

SK

When people are least sure, they are often most dogmatic.

— J. K. Galbraith

We often find ourselves becoming strident and aggressive without any apparent reason. We insult our colleagues, hurt our friends, frighten our children. We may think we are being strong and assertive, and yet the effects are just the opposite of what we intend. We are hurting, and so we lash out and wound others.

What are we hiding? Why are we feeling threatened, vulnerable, and weak? We usually strike out when we are hiding our needs and fears. We think if we attack, maybe we won't need to let anyone in. We may believe that if we let people in, they won't love us, because as addicts we feel unworthy and shameful.

It is the strong who are tolerant and charitable and forgiving. As we continue to grow in confidence and strength, we will find that we are able to be flexible, patient, and open with others.

Weakness and fear make me defensive and dogmatic. I am striving to be strong, open, tolerant, and loving.

PW

We live each day with special gifts that are a part of our very being, and life is a process of discovering and developing these God-given gifts within each one of us.

— *Jeanne Dixon*

As our recovery progresses, we discover ways to share ourselves with other people. We feel the desire to act on things we've learned and to apply them in our relationships. This way, we can pass on to others the awareness and knowledge we have been given.

This wonderful urge to take action should be followed, not resisted. A spiritual awakening is just that — an awakening of the spirit, which then seeks to be part of all life itself.

When we discover our talents, whatever they are, we will be true to them and look for opportunities to use them. The challenge of doing this lets such qualities as integrity, courage, self-discipline, and compassion rise to the surface, where they become part of our daily practice. The alignment of who we are on the outside with who we are on the inside is a priceless gift of recovery.

My recovery gives me great joy. I will share that joy with others today.

SK

April

Treat a work of art like a prince: let it speak to you first.

— *Arthur Schopenhauer*

Many of us have had times when we felt that we always have to have and give an opinion about everything right away. After a movie or a concert, for example, we may want to step right in with our comments and judgments. Often we "shoot from the hip," without thinking or being attentive to our feelings or the feelings of others.

This can be a way of warding off the experience, enclosing it within words. All of us have feared that we might be caught off guard and compelled to change or expand our own ideas. We've feared being too vulnerable!

Images, sounds, poems, and plays can cause us to open ourselves to the unfamiliar and the new, and if we are quiet and attentive, we can come to fresh insights and understandings. So, too, with people. If we are patient and willing to listen, we will always be learning and growing through contact with others.

The beauty and joy of life dwell within differences. I am learning to be open and attentive to what has not been part of my existence up to now, so that it may come to color and enhance my life.

PW

Faith is the subtle chain which binds us to the infinite.

— *Elizabeth Oakes Smith*

Surrendering ourselves to a Higher Power is a big step. As addicts, trust has not been one of our strong points. On top of that, Step Three says we surrender to the "care" of God. Feeling cared for — nurtured, trusted, listened to — may not feel familiar either. The idea of a Higher Power who actually cares for us can seem pretty foreign.

A starting place can be the idea of simply making a decision. When we do that, we will be shown the way to turn our will and life over to the care of God. Building a relationship with our Higher Power is like building any other relationship; it takes time, honesty, and faith. God doesn't require perfect faith, only our willingness. If we do our part, God will do the rest.

Faith is knowing that which is beyond knowledge and seeing that which is beyond sight.

SK

When you're down and out, something always turns up — and it's usually the noses of your friends.

— *Orson Welles*

Friends ought to stand by us in adversity, and many do so. But if our sex addiction becomes public knowledge, we may find ourselves isolated by the illness that has always made us feel alone. Friends drop away, lovers leave, children retreat into incomprehension.

Now we really need support. We know we cannot go it alone; we have been alone too long. We need the strength that comes from other people.

This is when we come to acknowledge the power of the group. Our program is based on the affection, strength, and caring of our fellow sufferers, many of whom have been in dark and lonely places too. They understand; they are our brothers and sisters in sickness and in health. They understand, and they do not condemn us; they have compassion that comes from fellowship in suffering. As we learn to trust them, we participate in a new communion of friendship that gives us strength and love.

I need support, and I am finding it through my program and in my group.

PW

Children have never been very good at listening to their elders, but they have never failed to imitate them.

– James Baldwin

There may be times when the shame and fear of the past intrudes on the present. We worry that our children may have been harmed by our addiction to sex. When the time comes to make amends to our children, we can trust we'll know the way to do that. We may or may not choose to tell our children we are sex addicts. We may or may not explain the past to them. But we must honestly face the consequences of our addiction on our children and commit ourselves to helping them heal.

With the help of our group and the Twelve Step program, we'll know what to do when the opportunity for healing presents itself. One recovering person said, "The day I started to recover, my child did too. My amend for the past is to make the present different."

God, please grant me the courage to face myself so that I can face my children.

SK

I never know how much of what I say is true.
— *Bette Midler*

Often I don't know if I am speaking or if it is my addiction. When I express a desire, how do I know it is coming from me or from my addiction? I am so used to being dishonest and warped in my feelings and how I express them that it's hard to tell who or where is the real me.

Of course it is never easy, even when sane and healthy, to say exactly what we mean and mean precisely what we say. We are complex mixtures of conscious and unconscious desires and motives — and language itself can be slippery, even treacherous.

This is all the more reason, then, to strive toward frank, open, honest exchange. It takes time, patience, and practice, especially if we have been in the warped state of our addiction for a long time. This is why we cannot go it alone; we need our Twelve Step program and our meetings so that we can learn together the difficult art of speaking our minds.

I am learning to tell the difference between truth and my addiction.

PW

I demolish my bridges behind me. Then one loses no time in looking behind when one should have quite enough to do looking ahead. Then there is no choice but forward.
— *Fridtjof Nansen*

In our recovery, our life of spiritual exploration, we burn all our bridges in the effort to leave our addiction behind. It takes courage to give up our old ways completely. One lure of sex addiction is its familiarity. Although living as an addict doesn't work for us, we know how it feels and sometimes we settle for that.

The world of recovery can seem like uncharted territory. Only the Twelve Steps, the experience, strength, and hope of others, and our Higher Power, can guide us. The risks seem great. What makes them worth taking is our realization that there is no other real choice. We go forward or, in some sense, we die. We need to trust that we can do it. In recovery we are truly explorers, and everything we discover will help others after us who want to recover from sex addiction.

I can see the rewards of my hard work every day as I change and grow.

SK

A good meal ought to begin with hunger.
— *French proverb*

Eating can be an art, entertainment, a social occasion, a ceremony, but it is best done when we are hungry. Then food serves its basic purpose which is to sustain life and help us grow. The same is true of sex. Its basis is desire, physical and mental desire, not sexual obsession or craving.

Our addiction often has little to do with the basic demands of desire and all too much to do with sex in the head. We don't feel sexual; we think obsessively about sex. We are often afraid of the physical side of sexual love, so we take refuge in fantasy, pornography, or anonymous forms of acting out. We flee from our real needs into the crooked byways of our fantasies and obsessions.

Our First Step back to sanity is the recognition that we are not using our minds but being exploited by the mental pictures that form our storehouse of memories and fantasies. Sex in the head rules us; as physical beings we are out of control.

We can get back to sanity and wholeness when we break with the past and turn to new sources of power, action, and love.

I will seek out new ways of relating to my sexuality as a living force within me.

PW

Many brave men lived before Agamemnon, but all unwept and unknown, they sleep in endless night, for they had no poets to sound their praises.

— Horace

A recovering person told this story at a meeting: "I was living in a city with a large population of homeless and poor. Each day it was painful to notice the contrast between the beautifully dressed, seemingly self-confident people, and the poor who shared the streets with them.

"One day I realized I could empathize with how those homeless people felt. I'd lived my whole life feeling I didn't belong, with no family I could turn to, and not knowing if I would survive another day in my addiction. The compassion I felt was a reminder to me not to form my opinions about people by how they look. It doesn't matter what people think they see in me, or anyone else. Each one of us is wounded. It's just that some wounds are on the inside instead of the outside."

Today I'll remember that we are all in this world together and for a purpose, no matter what the circumstances of our lives.

SK

*The winds and waves are always on the side
of the ablest navigators.*

— Edward Gibbon

Many people who have been sailing blame the weather for their misfortunes. "If only we'd had good winds." Or, "We'd have won the race if we hadn't been becalmed." Or, "I never feel sick, but..."

So it is with our lives when we are under the sway of our addiction. We blame fate, chance, our genes, the devil, our parents, other people — always looking outside ourselves for some element to account for our defects and our failures.

But the good navigator knows how to read the signs and make the weather work to help the boat and crew. So, too, we can learn to be attentive to our relationships with the outside world, working in harmony with what is around us. The world is not a hostile place; we can come to feel at home here. But first we must learn to live at peace with ourselves.

I know I needn't blame the world for my shortcomings. I am finding a harmony between my desires and reality as I learn to trust my relationship with the world.

PW

*When you don't feel yourself anything, I mean
part of anything, that's when you get scared.*
— *Lillian Hellman*

It is a cruel irony of sex addiction that what we desire — intimacy — is what we fear and believe ourselves incapable of. It is sad that being sexual, the act that should bring us closest to someone, instead isolates us. Yet intimacy in its truest sense, whether sexual or nonsexual, is what transcends loneliness. It is a uniquely human need.

Fortunately, we can learn how to be intimate. We can actually become new people, capable of giving and receiving in intimate relationships. All it takes to start is honesty and willingness. As we learn to love ourselves for who we are, we will become intimate with ourselves and with others. Then, our sexual experiences will become intimate as well.

I have a deep capacity for intimacy, and my recovery is teaching me how to love.

SK

I asked my father what "assertiveness train-ing" is. He said, "God knows, but whatever it is, it's bad news for me."

— Sue Townsend

The new and the unknown often strike us as "bad news," especially if they are associated with changes in our social roles and customs. Many of us are used to the status quo and don't want to have to deal with new systems or ways of relating, especially when our sexuality is involved.

But now in many societies, patterns are changing rapidly, especially with respect to roles and relation-ships. Many women are asserting themselves; many men are enjoying more nurturing roles. This can be a time of challenge and excitement if we are willing to reach out and test the new.

Often our fears about our sexuality hold us back from becoming involved in new social movements. Our ad-diction paralyzes us and makes us afraid of the unknown. But with courage and commitment to our recovery, we will develop an openness to change and new associations.

May this day be a time for thinking about new roles and relationships without fear and shame.

FW

The terrible beast that no one may
understand,
Came to my side, and put down his head in
love.

— Louise Rogan

There are times when it seems easier to give in to despair than to fight our way out of it. The trick is to catch ourselves before we become so depressed that we're incapable of acting. For starters, we can ask, What else am I feeling? Am I angry, sad, resentful, feeling sorry for myself? There may be real pain beneath our despair — pain that must be expressed so we can let go of it.

We can also take good care of ourselves. We can eat right, get some exercise, go to an extra meeting, and seek kind and understanding people. Talking through what's bothering us and asking for what we need are good antidotes to despair. Most of all, we can reach out for our Higher Power's consolation and strength.

We may feel unworthy or hopeless and too tired to care. We may believe that nothing matters. But things do matter. We matter. Life matters. We don't have to struggle with despair and depression alone. Our Higher Power and other people are with us.

I am grateful for the spark of hope within me that can never die. Things will get better.

SK

Education is not a product: mark, diploma, job, money—in that order; it is a process.
 — *Bel Kaufman*

Sometimes we think of education in terms of cash and security: we have got to learn this before we can achieve that status. We talk about learning as an investment and insurance, and we get mad if it doesn't pay off.

Some of us may think of the education in a Twelve Step program in similar terms: I've got to Step Eight, only four more to go and I'm cured, I'm happy, I'm free.

But education is a way of being in and viewing the world. It is a way, a path. It should be a journey, an adventure, an exploration of ourselves and our relationship with others in the world.

Our programs take place in time and they go on for the rest of our lives. Each Step is an affirmation of a certain way of being and needs to be repeated and related to every other Step indefinitely. Like life, this kind of education is continuous, open-ended, and enduring.

My program is an ongoing process that continues to open new ways of being and relating to the world.

PW

Yes, we love peace, but we are not willing to take wounds for it, as we are for war.
— *John Andrew Holmes*

When we are willing to face the impact of our sex addiction on our relationships, we are ready to begin making amends. We can take responsibility for the consequences of our actions, especially those that were sexual. Acknowledging that we have harmed other people through infidelity, harmful sexual practices, or broken trust takes courage. Repairing the damage directly and appropriately takes a heart open to a Higher Power's grace.

As our past heals through our recovery, we will see that facing reality comes more easily. Thus, the honesty needed in making amends also brings our relationships into the present. We will find our sanity restored by telling the truth to ourselves and, when possible, to the people from our past. Regardless of how the amend is made, or whether it's accepted, we will find peace once the effort is made.

God, my heart is open to You. I know that You will show me the best way to make amends.

SK

Experience has taught me this, that we undo ourselves by impatience. Misfortunes have their life and their limits, their sickness and their health.

— *Montaigne*

Our program isn't working. We are misunderstood. Nothing's going well at work. We just can't see it through. Why doesn't someone help us?

Impatience! We become fretful and blame others for our shortcomings.

Impatience! We lose touch with the tempo of life and our own particular rhythm.

Impatience! We are convinced our addiction will never cease tormenting us.

Let's slow down and get back in touch with life's movement. We know that all things have their season and their motion and their end. It may feel like winter now, but spring will come and then summer. Nothing remains static; everything changes and grows. There is a pattern to all life — including ours — if we are patient enough to discern it.

I need to slow down to get in touch with the rhythms of my life and life outside me.

PW

Tact is the intelligence of the heart.
— *Anonymous*

Making direct amends involves much more than a simple, "I'm sorry." Indeed, many of us have received an apology from someone who believed that just saying the words would erase a past full of hurt. Rather than peace, however, we have been left with a nagging feeling of incompleteness.

A real amend is the right one for the relationship. Through the willingness we show in making a list of who we have harmed, we come to know what the right amend is. If we write a letter or apologize, our personal involvement makes the amend genuine and sincere. We can also choose not to contact the other person, but to make a sincere silent apology, and turn it over to our Higher Power. If it's an old lover to whom we're making amends, we must consider the person's present life and whether there's a spouse involved.

In all cases, the best amend is to change our life so that today's actions will not cause harm and have to be added to our list of future amends.

I can feel good knowing that every day I am in recovery is a gentle amend for the past.

SK

We are adhering to life now with our last muscle—the heart.

— *Djuna Barnes*

We may think that strength has to do only with the body or the brain — pushing the car out of the snow or making a decision and sticking to it. We may pride ourselves on our brains and our sinews, but we tend to forget the muscle of the heart.

In our addiction we have become so oriented toward artificial means of stimulation that we have lost sight of honest, direct emotion. We haven't related directly to people and things. Instead, we've related to people and things obliquely, through images and fantasies. Pornography takes the richness and feeling of the world and freezes the heart out of it, turning the wholeness of human beings into deadly, fragmented images.

We can put the heart back into our lives by opening ourselves up to relating honestly and fearlessly with other people in our program. There we can feel safe and experiment with the expression of emotions long dammed up in us. There we can dare to be ourselves.

I am learning to trust my heart and am not afraid of its feelings and messages.

PW

In the important decisions, we should be governed, I think, by the deep inner needs of our nature.

— *Sigmund Freud*

We make decisions all the time, and every one, large or small, changes us. Since change is frightening, making a decision can be frightening too. We can make the process easier by asking ourselves the right questions: "Do I really want to do this?" "Will it benefit my life?" "Is it realistic?" Such questions help us know our true feelings, which are the most important part of any decision.

Wrong decisions are often made by focusing on external things: "If I do this, it will please my partner." "I'm doing it because I want excitement and intrigue." "I'm in it for the money." "I want the power and status." "Maybe I'm running away from something I don't want to face — but so what?"

As sex addicts, it is important for us to avoid impulsivity and all-or-nothing thinking. We can take our time, and talk our feelings through with our friends or our group, and try to see the bigger picture. If we are still unsure of the right thing to do, we can ask for our Higher Power's help, decide, and then trust the outcome.

The only wrong decision is one made for the wrong reasons.

SK

At the bottom of the modern man there is always a great thirst for self-forgetfulness, self-distraction...and therefore he turns away from all those problems and abysses which might recall to him his own nothingness.
— Henri Amiel

Do we rush around or slide off into the world of fantasy to distract ourselves from looking at ourselves too closely? Are we afraid that we might find nothing but our own...nothingness? Is our sexual acting out a misguided search for some kind of identity at any price?

Identity is not something given, once and for all. And perhaps there is never a fixed point at which we can say, "I am that." Life is process, upheaval, reversal, change, and a continuous process of becoming. If we are brave enough to welcome change and the pains it can cause, we may never have to fear the vertigo of nothingness or the madness of distraction that becomes self-destruction.

I ask for the courage to welcome change so that I may continue to participate in the energy of the life process.

PW

To see, we must stop being in the middle of the picture.

— *Satprem*

Seeing something from another person's point of view is an important spiritual awakening. That moment of understanding is a gift. We didn't expect it, but suddenly it's there. Our world grows larger because our view of that person changes. That, in turn, deepens our awareness and can deepen the relationship itself. Having someone take the risk of sharing him- or herself is precious because it shows that we have proven worthy of their trust.

It's a good feeling to feel the immediate connection that comes with understanding someone in a new way. We might experience compassion, love, or respect. One thing is sure: there is no room for the negative in a true moment of awakening.

Such gifts come because we have been willing to search for them, and for that we can give ourselves credit.

May God help me to be truly interested in other people and in who they are.

SK

God alone can finish.

— *John Ruskin*

We may have been brought up with the idea that we always had to finish something once begun — a meal, a painting, a piece of work, a letter. In many cases this went along with our notions of perfectionism: if something is going to be done, it must be done perfectly — the way Dad does it, or the teacher, or God. And so, especially if we liked to experiment a bit or dream, we felt we really didn't measure up.

But many of the greatest artists — Leonardo, Cézanne, Picasso — left work unfinished, as if to show the margin between impossible perfection and their own striving. What mattered was the effort and the process and the struggle. Each viewer of an unfinished picture could, by responding to the work's creative urging with her or his imagination, fulfill the process.

Our lives are never finished — at least until we can no longer add any final touches. We are always in a process of change and becoming. That is why we keep taking the Steps in our program over and over — to remind us that our lives are journeys, always in the act of unfolding.

I feel relaxed when I view my life as an ongoing creative process rather than as a perfect work of art.

PW

To live happily is an inward power of the soul.
— *Marcus Aurelius*

One person's joyous enjoyment of springtime may be another person's painful memories of a life somehow unfulfilled. One person's winter wonderland may be another's stark and hopeless landscape. One person's summer at the beach may be another's battle to avoid looking at people wearing hardly any clothes. One person's ripe and tranquil autumn may be another's sense of imminent death.

Each season of the year brings its own challenges. Many of us who are sex addicts feel sad or alone particularly during the spring and summer. All around us are people in love (not us) or people we think look happier than us. We may feel inadequate. So we struggle yet again with the same old feelings or memories.

We can remind ourselves that even though the past continues to resonate in our hearts, the present holds something different and better. If we open our eyes to the particular beauty of this season, we will be rewarded with its splendor.

I am willing to be open to this day's beauty and delight. The past is over.

SK

The purpose of freedom is to create it for others.
  — Bernard Malamud

If we are fortunate enough to enjoy freedom, we know we must be vigilant and protect it for ourselves. Freedom implies responsibility, and we willingly assume it because we know that in freedom we have the chance to grow and thrive. It gives us the opportunity to make the best of our lives.

We also need to be attentive to the privations and desires of others. There are many who are not free and who, like us, prize freedom above all else. How can we help them? What can we do?

Our Twelfth Step bids us to reach out to others and carry the message of our program to those who are in need. Sex addiction denies people the freedom to be fully themselves and fully alive. People cannot be free and sane if their lives are ruled by addiction. By carrying our program to others, we can help them return to sanity and growth and freedom.

I want to be free and help others find freedom from their addictive behavior.

PW

There is luxury in self-reproach. When we blame ourselves, we feel no one else has a right to blame us.

— *Oscar Wilde*

Just as we don't have the right to judge someone else, we don't have the right to judge ourselves. Our addictive script in the past was that when we did something we felt ashamed of, we judged ourselves guilty. All too often, we then punished ourselves.

Was that behavior an expression of our shame and sadness because we're sex addicts? Punishing ourselves won't stop the addiction; loving ourselves will.

We are grateful that our recovery has taught us the difference between guilt and shame. Guilt lets us feel remorse and sadness when our actions violate our values. Guilt helps us know when we've acted badly; shame tells us we are bad. Guilt gives us a way back to our selves through making amends; shame leaves us hopeless. To give in to shame and self-hatred only harms us and intensifies the power of the addiction. There is a better way, and that's to learn to love ourselves.

God, please step in when I feel the urge to take things out on myself. May Your love for me teach me to love myself instead.

SK

To be alive—is Power—
Existence—in itself—
Without a further function—
Omnipotence—Enough—
> *— Emily Dickinson*

It seems that as infants we longed for absolute power so that our pleasures would have no end. Always feeding, always in control, always contented. We were omnipotent and grandiose in our desires and our expectations.

This Pleasure Ego was in control of many of our acts as sex addicts. We sought to extend our enchanted empires and bend other people to our wills. We loved to look at bodies that were in thrall to our fantasies or our wills. We may still be willing to go to absurd lengths to get our way.

But recovery has taught us that simply being alive is a miracle and power enough. We learn to love the differences of other people. We don't need to prove our power at every moment, and we don't need to give in to our fear of being powerless.

By saying no to our selfish, grandiose child, and saying yes to the daily miracle of being here on earth, we experience ourselves as truly alive human beings.

I'm going to say yes to life and enjoy myself as a miracle of creation.

PW

Only by caring for and loving ourselves can we feel safe. Many fears are borne of self-loathing.

— *Anonymous*

The need to feel safe is primary within each of us. Without safety, life is frightening and overwhelming. Not feeling safe can even affect our will to live. Why go on when we feel alone in a hostile world?

As sex addicts who have been buffeted by our own and others' actions, we need to put feeling safe at the top of our priority list. Safety involves setting boundaries between ourselves and other people. It means having our needs met. It involves affirming that we are competent and that we are lovable. It also requires inviting our Higher Power into what has been the void of our life. We can't feel safe living in a void. We have to fill it with something meaningful, and the choices we make will determine whether we live or merely exist.

I am acknowledging my need for safety, and I am working to balance it with my desire for risk.

SK

I shall tell you a great secret, my friend. Do not wait for the last judgment, it takes place every day.

— *Albert Camus*

It is easy to hope that at some time in the future we may redeem ourselves by some great act of heroism or undergo a dramatic conversion. But in the meantime, all too often, it's business as usual. Too easily we can become used to our addictive behavior, and denying that our acting-out hasn't harmed anyone. . .except ourselves and those we love and who love and trust us. Deep down we knew we were judging ourselves and being judged. Now, each day, we can assess our actions and evaluate our behavior. In this way we learn how our sexual acting out has affected every part of our lives and our relationships.

It is time to change. The longer we wait, the more ingrained are our habits and ways of perceiving and deceiving. If we live a lie, we will be judged accordingly, by ourselves and those close to us. Our program teaches us that we can change and grow and move ahead into the openness and fullness of each new day.

I don't want to come to the end of my life wishing I had freed myself from my addiction. I am glad I have begun the process of change.

PW

We don't receive wisdom; we must discover it for ourselves after a journey that no one can take for us or spare us...
— Marcel Proust

Many of us have known people new to recovery who enter a Twelve Step program only to encounter an enormous crisis or difficulty. It's tempting at that point to question the mercurial nature of life, which sometimes inflicts blows when someone is already down. Difficulties do serve a purpose, though. It's often in such moments of struggle that people become aware of the reality of their life and begin to make difficult choices. It's also then that the fellowship of our recovery group shines, offering its collective experience, strength and hope to the addict in need.

Many of us have known someone who refused or was unable to hear the message being offered at our meetings. It takes wisdom, patience, and detachment to know when to reach out to someone, and how far to go. The respect we feel for that person's recovery process as well as the faith we have in our Higher Power and the Twelve Step program can help us do our part and then let go.

Life is a learning experience. I can learn the lesson of my life, but not someone else's.

SK

Only the wearer knows where the shoe pinches.
— *English proverb*

When we are in pain, it is we who know where it hurts. Other people may be ready with suggestions and advice, but we are the only ones who eventually can know what the matter is.

We are each a unique expression of humanity and we are the only ones who can live our lives. When we are stricken with addiction to compulsive sexual behavior, we know where it hurts and how much. While we may have to bear a lot of pain, we can identify where it hurts and start to do something about it. When this happens, it's possible for others to come to our aid later on.

This is true in our program. We know where the hurt is and we take the First Step. In doing so we turn to others who help us bear the pain and walk by our side on the open road to recovery.

I acknowledge pain and I can know what the cause is. I am willing to take the First Step for myself and find help from others.

PW

Everything has its wonders, even darkness and silence, and I learn, whatever state I may be in, therein to be content.

— *Helen Keller*

If we want to know how to work the program, all we have to do is look at our own life. With what are we dealing now? Is it abstinence or slips? Financial difficulties? Job problems, family problems, or physical illness?

Whatever we're going through can give us clues on how we can tailor the program to help meet our personal needs. Each day, we can decide what Step we need to work, or whether to call our sponsor, or whether we need to go to a meeting.

We can remember that external events merely parallel internal struggles. There is a deeper view of our lives emerging if we can only learn to read the signs. When there are no signs evident and all is darkness, that's when faith is necessary. It doesn't matter whether our life is falling apart; maybe it needs to. What matters is our faith that God is putting it back together. If we work the program day in and day out without worrying about the outcome, we will come through all right.

To be a grateful addict is to truly accept my particular struggles, including that I'm a recovering sex addict.

SK

May

*Only that action is just which does not harm
either party to a dispute.*

— Gandhi

We may find ourselves engaged in a dispute and
determined at all costs to impose our solution, even
though we know it may harm our opponent. We don't
really want a solution at all; we want revenge.

The desire to harm others may derive from feeling
that we have been hurt, as children perhaps. We may
have been neglected and misunderstood or even abused
and assaulted. So the world owes us something and we
mean to collect. We may even bear grudges against successful people, not because they have done us wrong,
but merely because they are successful.

We need to let our shame and sorrow out into the
clear light of day. By opening ourselves up to others,
we will surely find that we can defuse our anger and
our desire to hurt others. We can stand on an equal
footing with others and have no more need for resentment and revenge.

*I know that I am gradually getting rid of my secret shame
that causes me to act out of anger and vindictiveness.*

PW

It is not only the most difficult thing to know oneself, but also the most inconvenient one, too.
— *H. W. Shaw*

Sex addiction can be easy to hide from other people. We could delude ourselves that, since no one knows what we're doing, our actions aren't that bad. It's possible to live a double life: a healthy person some of the time, and a practicing addict at other times.

Unfortunately, it is often necessary to find ourselves in great pain or facing horrible consequences before we confront our behavior. Otherwise, the complex defense system we erect to "protect" our addiction also keeps us from learning the honesty we need to recover.

Sex addiction is cunning, baffling, and powerful. Rigorous honesty is important, especially in telling other people what we would rather keep hidden. It is usually the things we try to ignore that we are yearning to share and let go. We owe it to ourselves to be as honest as the program teaches us to be.

Higher Power, just for today, let me be honest. If I have slipped, let me admit it. If I feel remorseful about something in the past, let me tell someone and heal.

SK

Unextinguished laughter shakes the skies.
> — *Homer*

From the beginning of recorded literature, poets have sung of the glory of laughter. Being human means having the power to laugh, and as long as we are here, we will surely need and cherish that power.

Laughter can reconcile us with others and with the world. When we go to the theater, for example, we feel a bond with others as we laugh together at some piece of folly or a witty joke. Through our laughter we are brought closer to other people.

Addiction isolates and drives us into ourselves. We retreat from our common humanity into a single unhappy consciousness. Our world narrows and joy retreats. Laughter is shut out.

In our groups we rediscover the joy of belonging to a community. Laughter is one sign of that community, and as we join in, we feel our isolation fading and a new sense of love and belonging emerging.

I am rediscovering the joy of laughter that keeps me in touch with others.

PW

The human mind can bear plenty of reality,
but not too much unintermittent gloom.
— Margaret Drabble

Being an addict was a full-time job. It took much of our time and attention as well as most of our energy. Many of us worked hard honing our character defects and developing new rituals and ways to further our addiction. Our sexuality was used in the service of our addiction until, eventually, the high of being sexual took on an air of unreality.

When we make a serious commitment to recovery, our addict is unemployed. Bringing ourselves, step by painful step, back into reality is our new full-time commitment. Rediscovering a world filled with life and people instead of suffering and addiction is an awakening we experience with the eyes of a child. Finding a world where people live with integrity, help each other, and work to make life better, is one we had forgotten. But it does exist, and we're part of it now that we're in recovery.

Each day when I look around and see how good life can be, I can smile and say, "I could get used to this."

I will take some time today to slow down and enjoy life. My motto for today is Easy Does It.

SK

He that can't endure the bad, will not live to see the good.

— Yiddish proverb

Some messages from our culture seem like attempts to persuade us that life should be easy, fun, and profitable — morning, noon, and night. Otherwise we're led to believe that we are being cheated out of the "rights" promised to those born in a country of privilege and plenty.

We may have to relearn life's hard lesson that to prevail, we often need to persevere and endure. Images seduce us with promises of immediate gratification; fantasies beckon us to the quick fix. It's not surprising so many of us succumb to addiction; we're just not used to having to wait and strive for our rewards.

To work to be free of addictive behavior we have to change our way of thinking about the world. We may have to learn, perhaps for the first time, to do without, to be patient, and to defer our pleasures — to wait for what rewards there may be. At first we may feel cheated and betrayed, but then, as our program starts working, we will gain more enduring satisfaction rather than the fleeting, empty pleasures of our addiction.

I am learning to be patient and to persevere in a world that was not constructed just for me and my pleasures.

PW

Honor begets honor; trust begets trust; faith begets faith; and hope is the mainspring of life.
— Henry L. Stimson

If anything characterized the severity of our addiction to sex, it was hopelessness. How often had we tried to stop on our own, only to slip again into the shame of acting out? How often did we promise ourselves we would start over tomorrow, that today was hopeless and we might as well do whatever we wanted?

The problem was that we were trying to remove the addiction ourselves, relying on our willpower and intellect. We don't have to recover alone, and there is hope. There is a Higher Power — each of us can choose what we name it — who will straighten out the mess of our life and our sexual behavior. Of course, it would be nice if that happened right away, but as we become willing to wait, we find that the strength and hope that allows us to live today is there. Feeling hopeful gives us a place from which to start changing. It gives us a reason to care, to keep going, no matter how great the odds, and to start again if we stumble.

May I never lose hope that I can grow and change. Today, I will look around and see where there's hope in my life.

SK

Every great mistake has a halfway moment,
a split second when it can be recalled and
perhaps remedied.

— *Pearl S. Buck*

Sometimes we think we are driven on like sheep by the tyranny of our addiction. We may say that we were born sex addicts, that we were turned into sex addicts in our childhood, or that there's nothing we can do except to go on playing out our fate.

And yet, each time we are on the way to act out, there seems to be a second of clarity when we see what we are doing and where we are going. We feel a flash of freedom, and then, if we neglect it, the darkness of our addiction descends again, and we go onward to our "fate" like sleepwalkers.

Let's zero in on that flash of freedom. Each time we take advantage of it to change course and stop acting out, the light becomes brighter and the decision easier next time. We can take these small but sure steps away from our addiction and follow a new path illuminated by our freedom of choice.

I am determined to become more aware of my potential for acting freely in the face of my addiction.

PW

Self-love, my liege, is not so vile a sin as self-neglect.

— *William Shakespeare*

We will never achieve a feeling of true safety by seeing our self-image in terms of our character defects. To give our shortcomings such power is to ensure that we will never have enough faith or strength to go forward; we are either condemned to live in the past, trying to change it, or to the future, trying to control it.

The only safety is in the present, affirming the positive qualities we possess. Even if we're in deep sorrow this moment, we can feel safe by appreciating that we have the ability to grieve, which takes courage and passion for life. Appreciating our many good points is a way to counteract the fear that eats away at our security.

There are a number of ways we can affirm our worth. We can write affirmations, ask others for positive support, list our good qualities, and include our progress in recovery in our daily inventory. We deserve to have the freedom that comes from feeling safe within ourselves.

What am I saying to myself right now — "You're a failure" or "You're wonderful, and I love you"?

SK

Millions long for immortality who do not know what to do with themselves on a rainy Sunday afternoon.

— *Susan Ertz*

Many of us long to live forever. But when our addiction preoccupied us, we used to find time weighing heavily on our hands. We couldn't seem to get up and get going in the morning; there was a kind of sluggishness about us that comes from our self-concern.

Addiction made us self-absorbed. When we were thinking of our next high and the pleasures of tomorrow, we narrowed our vision until we only saw ourselves — and then perhaps we didn't like much what we saw. Our shame was in the foreground, blocking everything out.

Now, in recovery, we are learning to see beyond ourselves. If we are honest and work our program, we are coming to enjoy the present moment and yet see beyond. We need the larger view, and we are finding it.

I want to learn to see beyond myself and my pleasure as I expand my vision in the present.

PW

*Love of certainty is a demand for guarantees
in advance of action.*

— *John Dewey*

When we find ourselves wondering what we can do to bring our Higher Power into our life, let's remember that's not our job. Our Higher Power takes care of our conscious connection when the time is right. As addicts, we want to control everything, even the timing and manifestation of our Higher Power in our life. Luckily, it doesn't work that way — our Higher Power is not our codependent.

Our task is to work on willingness and openness, which is more than enough for one person. In the past, our willingness was based on a "What's in it for me?" system: "Tell me what I'll get from this, and maybe I'll do it." It was also based on control, which for many of us meant safety. Our willingness now comes from humility and a sincere desire to change. It shows faith in our recovery and in a Power greater and wiser than ourselves. To be willing is to surrender. I will Let Go and Let God.

God, I invite You into my life today. Please help me to be willing and open to You.

SK

The great end of life is not knowledge but action.

— *Thomas Huxley*

It is important to gain knowledge as we seek to understand ourselves and others. But we can also get caught up in insisting too much on knowing rather than doing. Maybe we are sometimes too introspective, too hooked on trying to figure everything out.

Often it helps to just get out there and do things. We may feel paralyzed and believe that we can only be "cured" when the moment of illumination arrives. But just undertaking little acts of kindness or daily tasks can set in motion a chain reaction that builds energy and self-confidence. Mend a fence, plant a tree, go for a walk with a friend. Yes, we *can* do it, and it feels good.

Love, too, is action. Love is not just a feeling but a connection, a reaching out, and a communion. Love is doing — doing things for others. At the end of the day, we may wish to write down not only what we have thought and felt, but what we have done — for ourselves and for others.

Let this be a day in which I set in motion loving actions that will help me and others.

PW

Don't hold the sprout against the seed. Don't hold this need against me.

— *Melanie*

Being human means having many different needs. Why, then, do we cling to the idea that we are totally self-sufficient, needing nothing and no one? Why do we treat our needs — physical, emotional, spiritual, intellectual — as mere nuisances that must be gotten out of the way as quickly as possible? Why do we keep pushing our needs away to the point of making ourselves ill?

With time, we will find the answers to these questions through a recovery program that substitutes gentleness for invulnerability, self-love for self-hate, and faith for fear. Once we let go of the delusion that all our needs can be met through sex and addiction, we begin to find out who we are and what we truly need. We will gradually let go of the fear that our needs will not be met, especially when we turn to other people. With patience and a realistic attitude, we will know the peace of having our needs fulfilled.

I live in the present, paying attention to my needs this moment and doing my best to meet them.

SK

The last time I saw him he was walking down
Lover's Lane holding his own hand.
— Fred Allen

Comic exaggeration startles us into thinking about ourselves in a new way. We can't really hold our own hand in an amorous manner, and yet we get the point.

Those of us whose sex lives were controlled by compulsions and obsessions often thought we were at least relating to our sex partners. But we may have been so focused on our own excitement that we hardly even saw the other person. Our own fantasy controlled our actions and dictated our pleasure. We lived in a world of our own.

Breaking free from sex addiction means breaking out of our self-centered ways of experiencing our sexuality. It means moving outward, taking risks, getting hurt, seeking the reality of other people, and learning to love. We may find ourselves holding hands — but with another mature, free, real, independent person.

I am getting tired of fantasizing about myself; my sexuality is an important way of exploring the reality of another person.

PW

What we don't know supports what we do know.

— *Bill Moyers*

There comes a time when we must turn and face our addiction. Running away will only bring terrible loneliness and isolation and intensify our pain. We must, instead, find the courage to face ourselves as sex addicts. We may believe we need our addiction to cover the feelings we don't want to face. Somehow, to admit that we have feelings and don't know what to do with them seems too shameful to bear. But to take the risk and discover that we can handle what comes our way gives us immediate strength.

It isn't easy to let ourselves experience our compulsion toward sex without surrendering to it. It takes a great deal of courage — courage we're never sure we have. The courage will be there, but often only as we're willing to reach out to our brothers and sisters in recovery in our moments of desperation. Courage doesn't mean doing it all alone. Meetings and phone calls are the lifeline connecting us; we need never suffer in isolation again.

If I am struggling with my addiction today, I will not run away. The addiction loses its power when met with the honesty and strength of the fellowship.

SK

*We have too many high sounding words and
too few actions that correspond with them.*
— *Abigail Adams*

It is easier to talk about what we are going to do than
to actually do it. We make good resolutions and can
use fine phrases to express our intentions. But when
it comes right down to it, we often fail to deliver.

Of course it is important to want to do good and to
talk about it. But if we get lost in our addiction, we will
find that the outside world tends to become shadowy
and insubstantial compared to our obsessions. I want
to buy him a present; I'd like to give her a surprise on
her birthday — but in the meantime, it's fantasy as usual.
In our addiction we don't have time or energy for other
people. Obsession takes time; compulsion costs money.
So the world must wait a while. . . .

In recovery we grow tired of living this way, so isolated and self-absorbed. It takes time, patience, and support to break out and start to live again, but we can do
it. We owe it to ourselves to turn good intentions into
results in the real world.

*I'm turning thoughts into actions and connecting with real,
live people.*

PW

I'm going to turn on the light, and we'll be two people in a room looking at each other and wondering why on earth we were afraid of the dark.

— *Gale Wilhelm*

Once we honestly acknowledge that our addiction to sex robbed us of our ability to be intimate, we are faced with the task of redefining intimacy and rethinking our attitudes and values about sex. Then we have to meet the challenge of restoring our sexuality to its rightful place in our life and forming intimate relationships.

There are many levels and kinds of intimacy. We used to think the only kind that mattered was sexual, but now we know we have a deep need to be intimate with ourselves, with God, with other people, and with life itself. Our part in being intimate is simple; it's the ability to relate appropriately to the circumstances at hand. If we're working, we do our best. If we're talking with someone, we give that person our full attention. If we're hungry, we eat healthily. Intimacy is participating fully, and in the present, in whatever it is we're doing. It means opening ourselves to all of our emotions, to joy, to reality. It means opening ourselves to life.

I can be intimate as much as I give myself wholeheartedly to the present.

SK

Who begins too much accomplishes little.
— German proverb

Some of us may feel that once we are on the road to recovery, we must complete our journey immediately, in giant strides. Either we are sick or we are healthy — there's nothing in between. So we must instantly, magically become perfectly sane and well.

We forget that a journey implies many steps, each one of which is complete in itself, and all of which have their meaning and value. Even our illness may have a purpose that we can't yet understand. Our recovery is a process whose design is only gradually revealed to us.

So let's not think we can wake up tomorrow totally cured; let's not take on the whole world all at once. Let's not seek to become perfect. We are all human beings on a journey that includes good and bad, right and wrong, failure as well as success. What matters is the journey and the striving toward the good.

I need to remember that I am human and on a journey that takes me forward one step at a time.

PW

I don't want my children coming up to me and saying, now what did you do, and me saying, I don't know.

— Dorothee Solle

Often, isolating ourselves disconnects us from the world until the only reality becomes addictive sex. When we isolate ourselves, time — an evening, a weekend, or longer — can slip by without us even being aware of it. Acting out also takes place in isolation; it doesn't matter whether we're with someone else or alone. The safety and connection we feel while acting out is an illusion.

When we become aware of our unhealthy actions, we must take care of ourselves, and quickly. The longer the isolation lasts, the more our awareness of it dims. If we can pick up the phone and tell someone else, "I'm isolating myself — I'm lonely — I'm afraid," we have made a tremendous start. To hear another voice, especially one that's caring, is to know we're not alone. We can be patient, giving ourselves time to learn how to be alone without slipping into isolation. The wall that keeps us apart from life cannot stand against our desire to be real.

I will live consciously.

SK

A poet begins in delight and ends in wisdom.
— *Robert Frost*

Artists deepen our sense of wonder because they have retained the ability to see life with a delighted eye. They know that nothing is too particular or minute to take pleasure in if we give ourselves time to pause and look. The world is infinite in its variety and beauty.

If we are addicted to sexual fantasy and acting out, we narrow our vision and see life with blinders. We are unable to relax and open ourselves to the new when we're so uptight and bent on our own pleasure. We are left impoverished.

We can learn, step by step, day by day, to slow down and really look at the world around us. We may find ourselves noticing the obvious things that we used to miss. This can lead to sheer delight when we notice that things can be so different, so particular in their shape, color, meaning, and impact. Delight can turn into knowledge as we explore further; then, if we persevere, we may stumble onto wisdom.

I intend to take time to pause and enjoy the world in all its particular richness and diversity.

PW

There are no precedents. You are the first You that ever was.

— *Christopher Morley*

We often compare ourselves to other people, and we usually come out poorly. We may not realize that what we're doing is harmful; we may think comparisons help us know ourselves better. "Her relationship is so good compared to mine." "He works the Steps better than I do." "She looks great; I look terrible." The comparisons go on and on.

Comparisons are an intellectual exercise, and as recovering men and women, we can put our intellects to better use. Security comes from an inner sense of self-acceptance, which grows every day we are in recovery. We will never discover who we are by comparing ourselves to anyone else. When we compare ourselves to others, we usually feel worse about ourselves. Comparing ourselves strips away our uniqueness and sets up a false standard we think we should meet. We are who we are. There is only one of each of us. We don't need to compare ourselves to anyone.

If I am comparing myself to others, I will remind myself that I am unique.

SK

Never forget what a man says to you when he is angry.

> — *Henry Ward Beecher*

Do we speak the truth when we are angry? We are always quick to say, "I really didn't mean it," and we may even try to make amends for our thoughtlessness. But people, especially children, rarely forget what was said to them in anger.

Angry words hurt and mark people. Even if our parents didn't really mean it, those angry voices and words are still with us. We often come to believe that our parents didn't love us or respect us; otherwise, how could they have said those angry things that still hurt?

We will always have moments of anger. But we can think twice before letting anger dictate our speech. Words can hurt and people remember.

I know I will sometimes feel angry, but I want to be sure that what I say is honest because people may take me at my word.

PW

And if by chance that special place that you've been dreaming of leads you to a lonely place, find your strength in love.
— *Michael Masser and Linda Creed*

Between disconnection and connection there is a time of transition. That time is called loneliness. During those moments, we choose what to do with that loneliness. We can stay in the lonely place as long as we need to; it's not necessary to force ourselves to move out of it before we're ready. But, eventually, we must move or the loneliness will deepen, becoming a desert of isolation where we cannot find our way out.

We are meant to be connected to many things: to God, to ourselves, to other people, to life. Maybe the purpose of loneliness is to provide the transition to connection. Rather than experiencing loneliness as something we deserve, or something we brought on ourselves, we can become aware of the deep longing within ourselves to be part of a wider world. We can then do our best to meet our needs and feel pleasure when they are met.

I will let my loneliness provide the impetus for moving me to a different place. I will be patient and gentle with my need for connection.

SK

If we all said to people's faces what we say behind one another's backs, society would be impossible.

— Balzac

In the program, to put our lives in order, we learn to be totally and fearlessly honest with ourselves. We lived so long and so deeply in the labyrinth of deception that we're no longer sure who we are and what we are about.

We have to live with other people. We need to get on with one another, and a certain amount of polite pretense is necessary. We need not hurt people's feelings simply to prove a point.

In our groups, however, we learn to be free to express our needs and desires to others without fear of blame or rejection. And at certain times we react to others honestly by giving tough, yet loving feedback. The group is a special place where openness and sincerity are the order of the day. It is a place where we grow by opening ourselves up to others, preparing ourselves for the kinds of intimate relationships that most of us are afraid of. And we carry a good deal of this honesty with us into the world.

I want to learn to be open and sincere with other people; I am learning to do that in the intimacy of my group.

PW

'Tis a gift to be simple, 'tis a gift to be free.
'Tis a gift to come round to where we ought
  to be.
And when we find a place that feels just right,
We will be in the valley of love and delight.
  — Appalachian folk song

We can take time today to feel our gratitude and joy. We know that our true self is emerging and becoming more present every day. For this we can be grateful. We are recovering from our addiction as we rebuild our self-esteem One Day at a Time. We know we are worthwhile and lovable, and for all this we can be grateful.

Just as we know joy, we have known sorrow, and we will know both again because that is the nature of life. But if we trust that our Higher Power is turning everything that happens to our good, we can truly say, "Thy will, not mine, be done." Is it asking the impossible to be grateful for everything that happens to us? Some days it may seem so, but those days pass, and after they do we sense their purpose in our life. It is then we feel content, knowing that we possess the promise as well as the reality of this new life we have chosen.

I am grateful for my recovery. I am also learning to be grateful for pain and difficulty because of the lessons I learn from them.

SK

I'd rather have roses on my table than diamonds on my neck.

— Emma Goldman

When we give gifts, we may think that if we don't give something extravagant, we've failed. It's diamonds or nothing. But we may be just using this as an excuse. We know we can't often afford diamonds, so we don't bother giving anything.

In giving, what matters is giving; the gift itself is a token of our affection, our caring. People like to know we are thinking of them and are concerned. Sometimes a card can bring as much joy as a necklace.

As we emerge from the isolation of our addiction, little acts of kindness and love become all the more meaningful in our lives. We need others to care about us and show their affection and concern. When we remember to think of others, we expand our awareness and stay in touch with the world beyond us. And that's what a big part of our new lives in recovery is all about.

I am a giving person able to show people I care about them.

PW

My inside, listen to me, the greatest spirit,
  the Teacher, is near,
wake up, wake up!
Oh, friend, I love you, think this over
  carefully! If you are in love,
then why are you asleep?

— *Anonymous*

We often know we have met a challenge in our life when we become suddenly aware of new knowledge. It's as if a light goes on, and things suddenly make sense. One recovering person referred to this as "a blinding flash of the obvious." It's important to take such a moment of awareness seriously; it is a cue that we have learned a lesson, and it's time to move on.

In the past, not trusting ourselves or a Higher Power, we relied on sex to make sense of our life. And the more we used our intellect and will to run our life, the less we accomplished.

In recovery, a moment of awareness is a moment of grace. It's as if our Higher Power gives us a wonderful gift, and we can say, "So that's what this is all about!" Our receptiveness to such a moment gives us the willingness to trust where we have been and the strength and courage to go where our life calls us next.

I will cherish the moments of awareness in my life today.

SK

An intimate truth is also a universal truth.
— *John Cournos*

Truth is often associated primarily with the larger issues and set alongside such ideals as Justice, Freedom, and Democracy. We like the grand words — and properly so on the grand occasions.

But let's remember, too, that truth between us and someone we are close to is also of supreme value. An endearment, a tender emotion shared, an admission, an apology, a vow, an act of forgiveness — all these take on the meaning of truth in an intimate context. And that, for all of us, is a context that matters.

How we are with one another on the level of feeling and trust is of vital importance. In building a meaningful relationship, we are implicitly making a statement about what the world can be — one built on courage, tolerance, affection, honesty, and love. Such truths as these will ring out clearly until the end of time.

I am uncovering many truths in my life that are connected to my relationships with other people.

PW

Come, Love! Sing On! Let me hear you sing
this song — for joy and laugh.
                    — Mechtild of Magdeburg

We have all known people whose lightness of spirit was a delight to us. That quality of "lightness" was expressed by one recovering sex addict in a dream she had where she floated to the ceiling of her room like a balloon. Letting go of our will and ego is a spiritual process that happens gradually. It results in a "lightness" that brings freedom to our lives and joy to others.

We can know we have lightened up if we see the humor in life. If we feel serene and don't care about having things our own way, we live with ease. Another person expressed it like this: "I was outside blowing bubbles with my daughter when I said, 'Look how they catch the light. The light is already there, all around, but it needs the bubbles to be seen.'"

I am the bubble; God is the light. To have a light spirit is to have a transparency that enables the spiritual to become visible.

Where is my spirituality? Am I in the realm of light? Today, I will let myself go to my Higher Power.

SK

Mere survival is an affliction. What is of interest is life, and the direction of that life.
— Guy Fregault

There are people who, when you ask them how they are, will say automatically, "I'm surviving." They say it with a bright, brave smile, as though they've battled tremendous odds and come through, bloody but un-bowed. Life is a grim, unfair business, they seem to imply. But in reality, their lives seem easy and secure.

Others with real problems — illness in the family, financial worries, job insecurity — might greet you with a smile and bring to the simplest exchange an energy and a liveliness that sends you away refreshed. Such people have the gift of life and share it abundantly. Like the ninety-seven-year-old woman with thirty-nine great-grandchildren who greets each one of them by name and has a story and a joke for every one of them. She lives in their memory as a force of love and vitality. Her immortality is there, in the love her family bears her.

Each day can bring as many joys as sorrows. When we are patient and find the courage to invest the best of ourselves, we can truly live rather than just survive.

I'm able to reach out and contribute to the richness of life. I can bring energy to those around me.

PW

Humor is emotional chaos remembered in tranquility.
— James Thurber

When was the last time something struck us as funny? If we see our life only in shades of black, we're probably being too intense. It may be difficult to find anything humorous about our self-defeating behaviors, but when we can, our recovery takes on a new dimension. To laugh at the pain we suffered from our addiction is not to minimize it, but to leave it behind. Laughing sometimes helps put our addiction in its proper place in our lives; it prevents us from giving it the mythic proportions it once had.

Lightening up and not taking everything — especially ourselves — so seriously is good for us. Instead, we can talk to a friend with whom we can laugh. We can choose a comedy instead of a tragedy. Whatever works. Our sense of humor is a special part of our personality; we can use it to detach ourselves for a moment from our problems. It will always help us stay in balance about life.

Go ahead — laugh it up.

SK

*All animals except man know that the ultimate
of life is to enjoy it.*

— *Samuel Butler*

If we take time to watch animals, we see that they have
a zest for life that seems to engage them totally in
whatever they are doing. A cat chasing its tail, a dog
going after a ball, a horse running along the shore, a
dolphin leaping and diving — all are actions that reveal
energy and delight in simply being alive.

Life, we say, is to be enjoyed, but how many of us
manage to put this theory into practice? We often associate pleasure with guilt or with acting out or with
hurting or being hurt, and so we stand back from the
full enjoyment of our power to be really alive.

Letting go of our shame and feelings of unworthiness
will help us to let go and live. If we can tap into the
spontaneity that runs through the animal kingdom, we
will rediscover the sheer joy of being alive.

---

*I'll try to take time to watch animals at play and learn from
their vitality and enjoyment.*

PW

June

*It isn't for the moment you are stuck that you
need courage, but for the long uphill climb back
to sanity and faith and security.*
— Anne Morrow Lindberg

It takes great courage to choose hope. It can seem so
much easier to simply give in to our addiction. Its
promises are so enticing — the lure of the next high
is just around the corner. We couldn't resist the sexual
pleasure held out to us while we were in the grip of
our addiction. After we acted out, it was even easier to
give in to hopelessness or despair. In the aftermath of
shame, loneliness, fear and self-hatred, it was hard to
find a way back to hope.

But there is a way back through the hope we find in
our Higher Power, and in the support of other group
members. An addict does not choose hope lightly —
there's too much at stake, and our hopes have been
dashed too many times. Within us, somewhere, is the
memory of who we really are and how good life can
be. Within us are buried feelings of happiness and freedom that we want to believe we'll feel again. We find
hope when we summon the courage to look for it.

---

*Am I feeling hopeless today? If so, I will rearrange my atti-
tude by claiming my power to make good choices. I will turn
to others willing to share their hope with me.*

SK

The worst sin towards our fellow creatures is not to hate them, but to be indifferent to them; that's the essence of inhumanity.
— *George Bernard Shaw*

Hate is the other side of love and shows at least energy and passion. Probably most of us feel surges of hate at some time or another, especially toward those we love the most. We can deal with this if we realize that these moments will pass and be forgiven.

But indifference and apathy can become a disease of the spirit so pervasive that their darkness envelops everything. Then life is stifled and throttled at the root. If we don't value the people around us, they will feel our lack of caring as striking at the heart of their humanity. If we have no time for life, then life and those close to us will drift away from us.

The world is a place of splendor and love. We can connect with it if we reach out beyond self-concern and replace indifference and apathy with the energy of living and loving.

Apathy maims and kills. I am discovering how to energize my body and spirit and reach out to others who need me as I need them.

PW

It is an old and ironic habit of human beings
to run faster when we have lost our way.
— Rollo May

Our boundaries are both inside and outside ourselves.
No one can set them for us; we can only set them. When
we come into recovery, boundaries are often unfamiliar.
We may wonder, What are they? How do we use them?
Many of us come from families where, as children, our
boundaries were disregarded, creating a pattern we continue to act on as adults.

Starting to set boundaries for ourselves takes time and
practice. Because the experience is unfamiliar, we may
often find ourselves veering between two extremes —
holding back for fear of blurring our boundaries or
acting as if we have no boundaries at all. But our willingness to set boundaries and stick with them brings us
a clearer sense of who we are. We begin to learn where
we start and end. We start to learn the same about other
people. With boundaries comes a new sense of self-
respect because they are our affirmation to ourselves
that we are not objects to be trampled on or used, but
we are human beings with dignity.

I know my own limits, and if I don't, I have every right to
learn them.

SK

Most people would rather get than give affection.
— *Aristotle*

Many of us who are sex addicts tend to be introspective and self-concerned. We are sensitive people whose affections may have been rejected or misinterpreted when we were young, so we turned to ourselves for the love we needed.

There is nothing wrong with needing love. Many people are afraid to admit this, because they fear rejection as soon as they make themselves vulnerable. Affection is necessary for growth and productive action in the world.

If we believe we are lovable, we will surely be loved. But we also need to love. We need to get out of ourselves and contemplate the characteristics of another person. Love is a two-way process, giving as well as receiving. We have to feel ourselves as really lovable before we can reach out to others. And we can learn to do this in our Twelve Step program. We can also learn, by listening to others and giving feedback, that it is good to give as well as receive. Being healthy again means we have rediscovered the power of love.

I am learning to see myself as lovable, and now I can tap into the energy that comes from reaching outward to others through love.

PW

She looks for me. God. Let her look for me and
tell me why she left me.
— Stephen Sondheim
George *in* Sunday in the Park
with George

To be left by someone we love is to experience a break in the heart's flow. To be left is to endure unanswered questions, to feel fear, anger, rejection, grief. It is life in the passive tense: we did not leave — we were left. Spiritual separation, when the bond of two spirits has been severed by someone else's choice, hurts badly. Where is the hope? How do we go on? At its most painful, being left even brings the question, "Do I want to go on?" Once we answer yes to this, we can start to heal.

We can choose to accept what is. We can find our way with the help of God's grace and the support of people who love us and want us in their lives. To yield to someone's wish to end a relationship is an act of respect. To want the best for someone, even when it means enduring our own loss, is an act of love.

Honestly grieving the loss of someone is a sign that I am already beginning to heal.

SK

Nothing in life is to be feared. It is only to be understood.

— *Marie Curie*

Fear usually comes from ignorance and it paralyzes usually only as long as we remain in the dark. For sex addicts, fear is often free-floating anxiety that overtakes us inexplicably and pushes us toward unaccountable actions.

Anxiety and fear have causes, and if we are brave enough we can explore them and put the bogeymen to rest. We can't always do it alone, though, because we need to hear some reaction to our insights and hunches about where our fear comes from. We can often find our true selves in the shared struggles of another person or in the words given back as we tell others about our fears and hopes. Most of us have been alone too long with our feelings trapped inside.

We are striving toward understanding, however long and painful the journey may be. We need to remember as we go that we are accompanied by good and loyal companions. Every step we take can be a yard won back from fear as we become familiar with the new and uncharted territory.

I will think and speak my way out of ignorance and fear, accepting the companionship of others along the way.

PW

I left because there was no room for me. But you could tell me not to go. Say it to me. Tell me not to go.

> — *Stephen Sondheim*
> Dot in Sunday in the Park
> with George

To leave someone we love is to knowingly break a vital connection. Even if we chose to leave, we wonder why it often hurts so much. But the heart isn't logical; it feels the trauma of the loss and the responsibility of being the one to say good-bye.

Love is a process; it doesn't end because we say good-bye. No matter how painful or harmful a relationship was, there were good things about it, just as there were lovable things about the other person. The challenge is to accept with grace the choice we've made and to forgive whatever hurt we've received. We can refuse to indulge in self-righteousness or indignation. Those feelings are born out of the illusion of power that comes with being the one who leaves. Most of all, we can grieve the loss and then let go of the person we loved so that we can heal.

I am having to break some relationships because it is healthier for my recovery. Still, I can hurt and grieve over the loss of those relationships.

SK

You grow up the first day you have the first real laugh—at yourself.

— Ethel Barrymore

Infants chuckle and gurgle and find the world amusing, but apparently they rarely laugh at themselves. Perhaps that's because they're still very much the lord and master of their world. Even when they see themselves in the mirror, tots are more likely to find themselves incredible than hilarious.

As we grow wiser we gain a sense of proportion about ourselves and our position in the universe. Just as the earth is not the center of the solar system, so we are just one of billions of people on our planet.

Can we smile at ourselves? Or are we always guarding our dignity or feeling fragile and vulnerable? A sense of humor means the ability to enjoy human foibles, even at our own expense. Having this kind of humor helps us to put others — and especially ourselves in relation to others — in perspective. Perhaps it is only when we've had a good laugh at ourselves for our imperfections that we can really begin to gain in stature. By keeping our importance in perspective, we learn to grow.

I can enjoy a good laugh — and will allow myself the freedom of a sense of humor, especially about myself.

FW

Healing is complex and mysterious. Sometimes it can happen only through the mystery of the wound itself.
— Allan Bozarth Campbell

One way to live our recovery is to be a wounded healer. This image, often used in spiritual work, expresses the wonderful contradiction found in the promise that no matter how far down the scale we have gone, we will see how our experience can benefit others. It is not in spite of, but because of how far down we have gone that we can reach out to those who still suffer.

As wounded healers, we have gone through experiences in our life that have resulted in personal transformation — a spiritual awakening. Because of our sex addiction and recovery, we now have a wisdom that we desire to share with others. And always, the opportunity to share in someone else's healing is as much a gift to us as it is to the other person.

We must never forget that our powerlessness was, and is, a wound. It is also the way to new power.

May I possess the simplicity, humility, and compassion of the wounded healer.

SK

Second thoughts are always wiser.
— *Euripides*

We may pride ourselves on being spontaneous; we may like to act on the spur of the moment; we may even enjoy the thrill of taking risks. And there is much to be said for acting in this way, without too much thought or self-criticism.

But such actions may be part of our addiction. Perhaps there are times when out of anger or hurt or frustration, we act on impulse and find ourselves back on the same old slide towards shame and even danger. We say "to heck with it, things couldn't be worse," and off we go to act out.

Let's resolve to sit back at such moments and think a while. Why not try to find out what we really want at these times of high intensity? Is the pleasure or the relief that we seek worth the hurt it may do to us and to those we love? Do we even *find* the pleasure that our fantasy bids us to seek?

When we think again, we discover that what we really want is to be at peace with ourselves and the world.

I am learning to reflect before acting to be sure it isn't my addiction that is making the decisions.

PW

We were brought up with the value that as we sow, so shall we reap. We discarded the idea that anything we did was its own reward.
— *Janet Harris*

How good it feels to have work to do that is satisfying, especially if our inability to work was a casualty of our addiction. In the past, getting sick often, having poor work habits, being involved sexually with co-workers or not doing meaningful work may have triggered our addiction and kept us trapped as a way to cope with our feelings of uselessness.

Our job now may not be our life's ambition, but there are many ways we can give it meaning. Rather than waste time in silent resentment, blame, or boredom, we can do our best and feel good about ourselves. We can let go of anger. We can have faith that, whether we're aware of it or not, our job today is contributing to what our Higher Power has in store for us. We can also take some step, no matter how small, toward doing the work we really want to do. Today and every day, our work will be easier if we take care of ourselves and our recovery — and we will feel serene.

If I find meaning in my work, my life will have meaning too.

SK

Change means movement, movement means friction, friction means heat, and heat means controversy.

— *Saul Alinsky*

We talk about wanting to change, to face up to our addiction, and our desire is real and genuine. But we must realize that change can continue to involve real pain for ourselves and others.

We were so comfortable for so long with our addiction! It had become our pacifier and our crutch. We wondered why we should bother to move forward and away from our world of ritual and fantasy and acting out.

But were we really at home there? What about our anger? Our remorse? Our feelings of hopelessness and despair? Our shame that caused us to shun intimacy and touch? Were we truly comfortable? Has change been so harsh in comparison with the misery of our addiction?

Even knowing there would be struggles and disagreements along the way, one day we cried, "Enough! I am powerless." We were ready, then, to face our struggles for a new, honest way of living.

I know that change will be hard, but I'm glad to join in the process of movement and growth which is life.

PW

*And when I see you happy, well, it sets my
  heart free.
I'd like to be as good a friend to you as you
  are to me.*

— *Joni Mitchell*

Friends are one of the greatest gifts of our recovery, and they come as a result of a life that's sane and manageable. It takes time and energy to make and keep good friends, but the rewards are worth it. To these special people we can gladly give our honesty, our fidelity, our trust, and our unconditional acceptance.

As friendship grows, we find ourselves more able to understand our friend's needs. Is there a child to be watched or a kitchen that needs cleaning? Can we listen empathetically, without judging, to whatever a friend is going through? When a friend is sick, are we ready to help out? Can we put aside our needs because a friend's need is greater at the moment than our own?

As our recovery helps us develop the skills it takes to be a good friend, we can let go and let our friend-ships develop naturally. Then, we will be able to trust the bond of love between our friends and us.

---

*I will call a friend today and let that person know how much
he or she means to me.*

SK

Judge people by their questions rather than by their answers.

— *Voltaire*

Addicts tend to be talkative people. For some of us, it may be that we've spent too long alone and are dying for company. At other times, we may have things to hide and we talk to cover up. Talking nonstop is one good way to avoid asking the hard questions. It can also keep us from really listening and providing thoughtful answers.

We all need to talk, but we also need to take time to be silent. In silence we can assess ourselves and our position in the world and examine the things we want and need to know.

Our programs give us the opportunity to sit and be quiet with ourselves and listen to others. When someone is explaining a Step or telling her or his story, we can learn simply by listening and formulating the questions we need to ask during the discussion. A good question is worth a thousand thoughtless words.

I will take time this week to be silent and think about what I've learned about myself and the people around me. This will enhance my recovery and service to others.

PW

*The last of the human freedoms — to choose
one's attitude in any given set of circumstances,
to choose one's own way.*

— Victor Frank

There are days when life in recovery seems like a bad play that we're unable to walk out on. It would be wonderful if, after we bottomed out, we started recovery and made nothing but progress for the rest of our lives. Recovery, however, isn't like that. It's a day at a time, a step at a time, a problem at a time. We struggle, sometimes with no idea of where we're going. We discover that our brothers and sisters in recovery are fallible, just as we are. Sometimes we want to throw up our hands and say, "Is this what recovery is like?"

The answer is yes and no. To learn to modify our unrealistic expectations, change our attitudes, and work humbly on our character defects teaches us how to live life beyond powerlessness. Yes, we will sometimes run out of patience with the process of recovery. But we can never go back to how we lived before; we know too much. We can feel the feelings, yes, but despair and give up for good? Never.

If today is a difficult day, I will still be hopeful. I'll act as if and have faith that things will get better.

SK

There's always an easy solution to every hu-
man problem — neat, plausible and wrong.
— H. L. Mencken

How can I recover from my addiction? What must I do to get well? These are the basic questions we ask ourselves as we struggle with our illness.

The questions are obvious, once we have taken the time to really think about what is going on in our lives. And the answers are just as simple — stop acting out, keep working the program.

But it's not enough just to come to meetings and put in time. Easy solutions may seem plausible, but just mouthing the words isn't going to do the job. We have been sick people, very sick at times, and we are going to need to struggle sometimes to see things straight again, to get back on course. The route is charted by our program and we have good counselors and friends as guides. But when all is said and done, we have to make the choice to accept the answers and help that will bring us renewal and health.

I know the way forward to health isn't easy, but I have con-
fidence in myself and in the program. I will come through.

PW

Life is judged with all the blindness of life itself.
— George Santayana

God may not always give us what we want, but we will always get what we need. Of course, in order for that to happen, we have to redefine the word "need." Our sex addiction led us to believe we needed more sex — a need that was insatiable. Along with sex, we may have been convinced we needed more money, more people in our lives, a better job, more clothes, and on and on. The list was endless because the needs were coming out of our addiction, which is never quenched.

As our recovery progresses, more of our true needs — those that enhance our life, such as hope, fellowship, and good health — are being met. We become willing to put in the effort and let go of the outcome. Most of all, we believe there is more than enough of everything we need. A life centered on our Higher Power stills the addictive hunger and takes away our shame at being people who need. We can never make up for the past, but we can live today with confidence in the generosity of life.

In recovery, I'm able to tell the difference between my needs and my greed. I can meet my needs without worrying there will never be enough.

SK

What is the use of running when we are not on the right road?

— *German proverb*

We charge through life, many of us, at top speed, thinking only of our performance and our goals. We may be moving so fast because we don't want to slow down and take a good, hard look at the road we're on and the kinds of things we're doing.

Speed kills, and not only when we're driving a car. Speed can kill when we are driving ourselves beyond our limits. Excessive speed is bad for our mental and physical health.

Let's slow down. Why not take time each day or at least a few times a month to sit around and do nothing? We can learn to look more closely at the world if we're not moving so fast. If we give ourselves time to be in touch with our loved ones, we will notice all kinds of things that up to now have passed us by. Let's make sure the road we're on is the right one for us.

After all, life isn't a race, it's a journey.

I see, hear, touch, taste, and smell things more fully as I take the time to relax and be attentive to everything that is on my path.

PW

"Men have forgotten this truth," said the fox. "But you must not forget it. You become responsible, forever, for what you have tamed. You are responsible for your rose. . . ."
— Antoine de Saint-Exupery

A recovering person once spoke about responsibility and said that, for her, the challenge is "respond-ability," how to respond to what life asks of her.

Responsibility can be a frightening word; perhaps we thought of it as a synonym for failure. How many times was irresponsibility the norm when we were giving our energy to our sex addiction? Behavior such as revolving-door relationships, "forgetting" about birth control, infidelity, and frequenting potentially dangerous places, were all signs of irresponsibility. Life as an addict was a treadmill, and we couldn't get off.

When we assume responsibility for our thoughts, feelings, choices, and actions, we truly grow up. We can meet the challenge of responsibility by not expecting perfection. We can examine our options before we make choices and learn to enjoy our life. It is then we will experience manageability and sanity — gifts of recovery.

Today, I will choose to be responsible by responding to my needs.

SK

We are confronted by a condition, not a theory.
— *Grover Cleveland*

By and large, our present age invests heavily in the idea of introspection. We like psychological theories and think we are on the way to discovering what makes people tick. In the area of sex, especially, we have high hopes that we will soon get it all figured out and solve the enigmas that baffled Oedipus and Freud.

But sex is not just theory any more than life is. It's there, in all of us, every day — a force, a feeling, part of us. In our case, it's out of control; as recovering sex addicts, we are just learning how to manage this vital part of ourselves.

Will theory help? Up to a point. We can try and figure out the origin and causes of our actions. But understanding needs to be doubled by action: we need to take steps to reorient our behavior. That is why our program has action Steps at its core; we are on the way, continuously, to change and renewal. We never arrive at a point where we can say, "Ah, yes, I understand that now; it is finished." That would be too neat and, in a way, an insult to the glorious complexity of sex and life.

I am moving through life, moving and growing as a participant in the human condition.

It is not only for an exterior show or ostentation that our soul must play her part, but inwardly within ourselves, where no eyes shine but ours.

— *Montaigne*

One of the first things we learn in recovery is that we have choices. This can be a startling realization, for as sex addicts we gave our lives over to the comforting delusion that we had no choices, that we were victims of life.

We face many choices during the day. In fact, everything we do is a choice. We may think the small choices — what to wear, what to eat, whether to have coffee or tea, whether to go to a meeting — are unimportant, but together they make up the fabric of our lives. It is those choices, made one at a time, that we lean on when we have to make big choices. And our ability to be abstinent, the most important choice of all, is determined by the small choices we've made out of love for ourselves and commitment to our recovery. We can be grateful that recovery has restored to us the power of choice.

I may be powerless over my addiction, but I'm not helpless. I can make choices.

SK

*Every child is an artist. The problem is how
to remain an artist when you grow up.*
 — *Picasso*

To be an artist is to be tuned in to and turned toward
the new, saying yes to life in all its diversity and richness. Healthy children face life with openness and
creativity. They make things, play make-believe and
create a world of beauty and delight.

We are still children if we dare to welcome the creative force within us and relate it back to the spontaneity
and newness of our childhood. There may be shadows
and even darkness to overcome, but if we are brave we
can rediscover that childlike energy and freshness.

Picasso went on creating for over ninety years. He kept
the child alive in himself for our delight. Even if we do
not have his talent, we can be inspired by his example
— to bring to life the creative child in us again.

*I am glad to be getting in touch with the creative child who
is still alive within me.*

PW

Weeping may endure for a night, but joy cometh in the morning.

— *Ps. 30:5*

It's important to know we are not to blame if we didn't learn when we were children what we needed to know about sexuality, relationships, and living a healthy life. It's not a child's job to teach him- or herself what is needed to live happily.

While it is difficult as an adult to learn the things we should have learned as children and adolescents, it is not impossible. We can rely on the courage, strength, and humility we show by being willing to live in recovery One Day at a Time. We can also ask our Higher Power to help us develop our spirituality, which gives us the inner truth we need to live. We may feel angry sometimes, or get tired of struggling, but we must have faith that we can do it. The yearning within us to have relationships and to contribute our skills and talents must become reality. Continuing to grow gives us a sense of accomplishment and a wider world that is ours to experience.

Today, I will feel proud of my ability to take risks in order to enlarge my life.

SK

A fellow-feeling makes one wondrous kind.
— David Garrick

Anonymous or loveless sexual encounters left most of us untouched by any genuine human warmth. We came away from them not enriched but impoverished, and gradually our lives became grey and cold and hopeless.

Sex can be lonely, scary, and sad if it isn't enfolded in affection. We would become vulnerable if we gave ourselves without love. We could even become heartless and cruel, seeking our own pleasure and satisfaction at the expense of other people. Our partners would not be partners at all, just objects.

Feeling for others, sympathy, affection, empathy — these are the human emotions we need to cultivate alongside our sexuality. And we learn to do this in our program. Sex needs to be encompassed by feelings of caring and tenderness; we need to be held and looked at and loved in order to feel secure. Sex can be frightening, but love contains and banishes fear.

I want to be kind and loving and relate to people with my whole self.

PW

We find rest in those we love, and we provide a resting place in ourselves for those who love us.

— St. Bernard of Clairvaux

How wonderful it is to feel that we belong! This is the security that comes as we gradually look outside ourselves and connect with other people. As we break free of the isolation of sex addiction and give up such self-defeating attitudes as being fearful and resentful, we find a new ability to be out in the world.

We can go to work and feel that we're part of a group. We can walk into a restaurant and know we belong there, and not feel that everyone is looking at us. We can go to a meeting and experience the wonderful sense of community that only comes from being with other recovering sex addicts. We can do volunteer work, join a church, or go out with a group of friends. And in all of these activities, we discover that we not only get to know others, but we let them get to know us as well. Believing that we belong is a gift that comes from our ability to be ourselves, no matter what the circumstances.

I believe that I belong. No matter where I am or what I'm doing, I have something to contribute.

SK

Humankind cannot bear very much reality.
— *T. S. Eliot*

Most of us who are sex addicts are all too ready to turn our backs on reality and take refuge in fantasy when the going gets tough. If we suffer a setback we tend to run away to revise it in our minds. If our feelings are hurt by a lover, perhaps we turn to pornography or a meaningless affair to get cheap and nasty revenge.

In our addiction we sustain our fantasy world and extend our childish dreams of omnipotence. There we are all-powerful and our sexual gratification knows no bounds. Other people become marionettes who dance on strings to the tunes we call. Reality is a distant smudge on the horizon.

In recovery we learn to bear the discontents and disappointments that come our way without having to leap back into fantasy. By listening and talking we anchor ourselves in a community that is not afraid of life. Here, in our groups, we develop a steadier gaze and a firmer grip on reason. Reality may be harsh at times, but it is also joyous and fulfilling, and now we can cope. We can enjoy the bright, fine moments, and bear misfortune with good grace.

I am learning to look at life steadily and go forward without plunging into fantasy in order to solve my problems.

A natural pleasure is one thing; an unnatural pleasure, forced upon the satiated mind, is quite another.

— *Thomas Merton*

All around us we come in contact with advertising, movies, music, music videos, TV, books, and magazines that use sex to sell a lifestyle or a product. The news is full of stories about pornography and child molestation; our instincts tell us this is sex addiction, although the news never explains it that way.

How do we keep ourselves and our recovery safe in a world where sex addiction is called every name but that? How do we maintain our reality in the midst of society's denial? How do we stay abstinent when our culture often encourages us to act out?

We must be fiercely protective of our recovery and rigorously honest. We are responsible for knowing what triggers our addiction and for staying away from persons, places, and things that might do that. We do not have to worry about educating the world or trying to change it. We have chosen to live another way, safe within our spirituality and our program of recovery.

God, please help me detach from the world's preoccupation with sex, and help me stay true to my abstinence.

SK

The best mask for demoralization is daring.
— *Lucan*

As sex addicts we know what it feels like to be demoralized. Our addiction caused us to lose sight of our moral values, our beliefs, and our spirituality. We fell into mechanical patterns of fantasy and acting out that were separate and isolated from our deepest sense of morality and values.

The way out is by finding the courage to reassert our connection with others and our relationship with our Higher Power — in a word, through the rediscovery of our spirituality.

Sex addiction thrives on shame and isolation, and it withers in the light of openness and honest exchange. In our program we talk with others, follow the Steps, assess our progress, and dare to be free. We thus find the courage to overcome our demoralization.

I want to dare to be open and honest with myself and with others.

FW

Every adult is in need of help, of warmth, of protection, in many ways differing from and yet similar to the needs of the child.
— Erich Fromm

A common thread in many sex addict stories is childhood sexual, physical, emotional, or verbal abuse. Abuse is a powerful force against which a child is helpless. Eventually, it can make a person vulnerable to sex addiction and other addictive behavior.

That's why it's imperative now that we treat ourselves lovingly. Only in this way will the healing force of recovery take hold in our hearts. Just as we wouldn't rub sand in a wound that is healing, we cannot continue the patterns and habits of the past. The child within us who still hurts deserves all our care and our unconditional love. When we lapse into self-pity, blaming, rage, or resentment, it may be a clue that our addiction is in motion. The feelings that are causing us pain need to come to the surface so we can express them and be comforted. Saying the Serenity Prayer or making a phone call can restore our hope and give us the strength to turn away from old behavior.

What am I saying to myself right now? I will talk to myself in the same caring way I want others to talk to me.

SK

I have never known any distress that an hour's reading did not relieve.

— *Montaigne*

One of our tools of recovery is reading. Most of our groups have daily meditation books from which we read aloud, and many of us read a meditation each day at home. We find that the writing, short and compressed, helps us to collect our thoughts, and then our minds and feelings expand outward beyond our reading.

Reading is not only entertainment; it is a kind of silent conversation with ourselves. And as we browse through our favorite books, we carry on a dialogue with old friends. We are taken out of ourselves and moved more deeply into the process of living.

As sex addicts, we need this. Most of us are often locked away in our worlds of fantasy and fear. We need the kind of intimacy that can come from reading, and we need the interaction and stimulus that inspiring books give us. We can move out and talk about them with our friends and enlarge our circle of knowledge and experience.

I'm grateful for the opportunity to read, which takes me out of myself.

PW

July

*My life is. . .a mystery which I do not attempt
to really understand, as though I were led by
the hand in a night where I see nothing, but
can fully depend on the Love and Protection
of Him Who guides me.*

— Thomas Merton

There are many different ways to express spirituality,
and I know that my Higher Power is showing me my
way. Spirituality is not necessarily religion. It is the
yearning of the heart toward God, the desire to leap the
chasm that divides us from the infinite and eternal.

For some, spiritual expression is a shout of gratitude
and praise. For others, it's a journey through a desert,
darkness, or a frozen landscape. For still others, it's a
search that happens unconsciously, without their really
being aware of it. As recovering sex addicts whose
progress depends on a spiritual life lived a day at a time,
we must be true to our own spirituality. We must trust
it, no matter how difficult the journey. Nothing is too
great for God's unconditional love—not sex addiction,
not fear, not unwillingness. Only our happiness matters to the God who loves us, who led us into recovery
and into a new life.

*When I laugh, God laughs. When I weep, God weeps. When
I need, God says yes.*

SK

*It's not that I'm afraid to die, I just don't want
to be there when it happens.*
— *Woody Allen*

Many of us think of death in the abstract, as a fact
rather than a reality. We know that everything passes
and that we are bound to die, but we rarely allow ourselves to accept the reality of dying and being dead.

Perhaps our acting out is a way of avoiding the reality
of death. It may be that we can only think of sex as a
new beginning, a false sense of perpetual renewal, even
a kind of rebirth. Especially in fantasy and maybe in
our relationships, we are always "falling in love" all over
again. Always young, always beginning again, always
keeping our options open. Never settling into the con-
tentment of a commitment.

As we begin to mature in our recovery, we can learn
to integrate our thinking and feelings about death into
our feelings about our sexuality and our daily lives. We
can sense death as an integral part of life, and not just
as an abstract finality. This can become part of our
program, part of the process of learning to experience
reality in all its stunning diversity. Life can become more
precious as we realize that we must leave it.

---

*I am discovering how to explore my feelings about death
and integrate them into my process of recovery.*

The real sin against life is to destroy beauty, even one's own — even more one's own, for that has been put in our care, and we are responsible for its well-being.
— *Katherine Anne Porter*

A good way to start each day is by asking, "What can I do to take care of myself today?" To ask and answer that question is to affirm our belief that we're worth taking care of. It also requires looking within ourselves with honesty. Is it hard to admit we're struggling with our addiction? Or that we're feeling sick? Or that such feelings as rage, sorrow, or fear are predominant? Or that we're working through incest, sexual, physical, or emotional abuse issues?

Meeting our needs with gentleness and compassion softens the task of being good to ourselves. It may take a long time of asking, "What can I do to take care of myself?" before we actually know how to or want to. But just as a good parent thinks of how to take care of his or her child, we can learn to do the same for ourselves. Each time we do, we move closer to higher self-esteem.

What can I do to take care of myself today?

SK

Human misery must somewhere have a stop:
There is no wind that always blows a storm.
                                        — Euripides

It is easy to think we will always be in the same boat, that our characters are fixed, our habits unalterable. "This is who I am. You can take me or leave me." When we say that, we often really mean: "When you know who I really am, you *will* leave me." This is the ultimate position of the sex addict.

But no one is predestined to be a certain person or to behave in a particular way. And no one stops growing and changing. We have to have faith in the immense possibilities of movement and growth.

Life itself is more than winds and storms. It can be calm, changeable, hot, dry, mellow, promising, gloomy, bright, and serene, and we can match its immense diversity of moods. For we are part of life, part of all this wondrous change and diversity, and if we are not afraid to let ourselves go, we can be as varied and as flexible as life.

I don't believe that I am fixed in my ways or stuck in my addiction. I am learning to be open to all the changes that life can offer.

PW

O Body swayed to music,
O brightening glance
How can we know the dancer
from the dance?

— W. B. Yeats

Sexuality is not something we do, but it's part of who we are. We are physical, intellectual, emotional, sexual, and spiritual people, and all parts are equally important. To consider sexuality as energy, a state of being, rather than a state of activity, helps us put it back within ourselves as part of our healing and recovery.

Part of our challenge as recovering people is to explore what healthy sexuality is and to decide what our values regarding our behavior are. We are responsible only for taking care of ourselves; it is not up to us to decide sexual issues for others or for society. It is more than enough to know our own needs and how we will meet them. We can give ourselves permission to put sexuality in its rightful place. It is an important part of who we are, but only a part and not the whole.

My sexuality is an expression of my spirituality, a part of myself I nurture and love.

SK

*I was much farther out than you thought
And not waving but drowning.*
— *Stevie Smith*

Sometimes we misread the signs that our friends send to us. When we think they are cheerful and getting by, they may really be struggling and hurting. Especially if we are absorbed by our own lives, we may miss the subtle calls for help sent out by our loved ones.

This is particularly true if we are sex addicts. Our disease can throw us back into ourselves and cut us off from the lives of others. When we have sex, we often do not make love and spread joy; we go deeper into ourselves, into the darkness of isolation. Our shame and fear increase along with our loneliness.

We need to break out of ourselves and open our eyes to the distress signals sent out by others. As we reach out to help, our lives become richer and stronger. We gain immeasurably through connecting with others. Soon we will find the layers of our addiction falling away like an old skin.

I can learn to be attentive to other people and their calls for help.

FW

Prayer is our humble answer to the inconceivable surprise of living.
— *Abraham Heschel*

There are many ways to pray, and each of us has a style that uniquely expresses our spirituality. Once we open ourselves to our Higher Power, we can get comfortable with our own way of praying. It may mean leaving past ways behind. Maybe we've been used to prayer that relied only on words. Perhaps we used to pray for what we wanted, making sure we told God precisely what was best for us and everybody else. Or maybe we didn't pray at all because we didn't know how to or were afraid.

We need not worry about *how* to pray; our Higher Power shows us how. We must, however, be willing to move from the everyday world to a place where it is just our Higher Power and us. It is an exciting part of our spiritual journey to develop new ways to pray, trusting our relationship with our Higher Power to deepen the experience. What matters is that we give ourselves to it. When our prayer is from the heart, we know it and are at peace.

Prayer is *another word for "conscious contact with God as* we understood Him," *which is important to my recovery. I'll take time today to pray.*

SK

Wisdom rises upon the ruins of folly.
— *Thomas Fuller*

We gain *knowledge* from other people, but *wisdom* comes from within. We have to live our own lives, profit from our blunders, and learn from our experience. Nobody can do these things for us.

Part of living is making mistakes. And some of us have to keep on making the same mistakes until we suddenly make a breakthrough and achieve a new perspective on ourselves and our actions. It often seems we are never going to be ready for the next step — and then suddenly we take it and we come through. We think we're not going to make it; then we make a leap forward.

Nothing needs to be lost or wasted in our lives. Even the folly of our addiction can teach us hard lessons if we are attentive and brave. Our craziness may help us to see more clearly and gain insight into ourselves and others.

I can use my experience and mistakes to find wisdom and peace.

FW

A lie would make no sense unless the truth were felt to be dangerous.

— Carl Jung

It is risky to be rigorously honest with other people; it takes practice. It is also difficult to become honest with ourselves. Until we do that, it is almost impossible to be honest with someone else. As sex addicts, we must face the reality that even the smallest lie harms our recovery and can trigger our addiction.

Through working the Twelve Steps, we can learn the power of honesty and how to reject the fear, shame, or grandiosity that held us in bondage to dishonesty. We can use the Twelve Steps to restore to us our honesty and integrity. With our integrity back, nothing can happen that's as painful as the inner knowledge that we've been dishonest.

In recovery, we learn to be safe in the truth. As long as we remember how it used to be — the lies, the double life, the fantasies we thought were reality, and the impact of our lies on other people — we will find the courage and simplicity to be honest.

Which Step do I need to take today in my journey toward honesty?

SK

Anonymity represents to most people a liberating even more than a threatening phenomenon.
— *Harvey Cox*

When we join a group for sex addicts, we make a promise to respect the confidentiality of each and every member. We call one another by our first names, and we don't gossip about the social lives of our brothers and sisters in recovery.

Our groups act anonymously. We have no leaders, no spokespersons, no political affiliations. We meet and act on the basis of all for one and one for all.

When we talk in our groups, we can let go of our social identity and reveal the real human being beneath. Each of us is a unique person, but we share the sickness of sexual addiction that goes beyond the individual and links us to one another in our common suffering. Even though we may not know one another on a social level, we understand and sympathize and love one another as women and men journeying together on the road to recovery. I come to know you and you come to know me in a way that few, if any, other people know us. Anonymity allows us to be intensely personal and yet secure and unafraid.

I am glad that I can let go in the anonymous haven of our group meetings.

PW

Every day in every way, I'm getting better and better.

— *Emily Cove*

One of the insidious beliefs underlying sex addiction is that we can have an enduring relationship if we just find the right person. Many of us have treated people who have fallen short of our ideal of the "right person" poorly and we congratulated ourselves on our high standards, for not compromising. Others of us have reveled in the melancholic high of never having found the perfect soul mate with whom we could spend our lives.

We learn in recovery that we must let go of the idea that there is one perfect person. When we learn to love ourselves, and we give ourselves enough time to grow, we discover that our obsession with finding the "right person" fades. We may even be pleasantly surprised to find out that having a primary relationship is no longer a condition for our happiness. Although it can be lonely living without the primary relationship we want so much, our Higher Power gives us the grace we need to sustain ourselves until the time comes for us to be with someone, or until we've accepted it wasn't meant to be.

I will be patient with my heart's longings, loving myself and the people in my life today.

SK

Beauty is the promise of happiness.
                    — *Stendhal*

Often we are too busy or self-absorbed to notice what is beautiful in people and in the world around us. We hurry along focused on ourselves, inattentive to what really makes life worth living.

The world is filled with beauty — twilight over a lake, a child's laughter, a scene in a movie, the sun on a stone wall, a weeping willow, a lively song, our beloved's face. If we are attentive and learn to slow down, we will see all around us signs of beauty that speak directly to us.

We do not have to go to exotic places to find beauty. It is here, in our lives, all around us. Finding it, we carry it with us, and our lives are enriched. The language of beauty is the language of joy.

As I become more attentive to the beauty that is all around me, I find my life becoming happier and more deeply spiritual.

PW

*It is better to be lost than to be saved all alone.
It is, besides, an illusion to suppose that is
possible, when everything proves the solidarity
of individuals.*

— *Amiel*

Admitting we are sex addicts is recognizing that we
are suffering from much more than a bad habit we can
control if we just work a little harder. To be a practicing sex addict is to be powerless and to have an unmanageable life. It is to be obsessed with sex, however
we act that out. It is to lie to ourselves and others. It
is to be out of touch with who we really are. And, most
painfully, to be a sex addict is to be unwilling to give
the addiction up.

Once we surrender to the reality of sex addiction, we
can begin to surrender to the reality of recovery. We
simply have to admit our powerlessness and unmanageability. We do it alone; no one can do it for us. But it
is the last thing we will do alone. From now on, we will
have our recovery program, the fellowship of our
recovering brothers and sisters, and our Higher Power.
We will never be alone again.

*Though admitting powerlessness can cause me to be fear-
ful, it can also cause me to grow. This growth is essential
for my recovery.*

SK

*I complained because I had no shoes until I
met a man who had no feet.*
— *Persian proverb*

When we are locked away in the loneliness and self-pity that comes with our addiction, we often exaggerate our misfortunes. In our solitude we feel we are unique in our troubles and unhappiness, and that there's no way out.

But if we open our minds and hearts, we will find that there are many people whose lives are filled with real hardship and pain. Yet, many of them manage to be cheerful and loving. They may be poor, handicapped, or bereaved, but they daily show courage and have serenity in their lives.

In our groups, too, we meet many whose lives have been blasted at the root by neglect, abandonment, or abuse. And yet they have left behind bitterness and anger and grown into healthy, kind people. When they take time for others, they give us some of their courage and affection.

Our lives can become richer as we realize our good fortune at being in recovery with brave and kind people.

I'll remember to give thanks to the people in my life who nourish my health and my spiritual development.

PW

The spiritual life springs forth in the pastures
of the heart, in its free spaces, as soon as
these two mysterious beings, God and man,
meet there.

— *Paul Evdokimov*

Sex addiction is a spiritual disease. Living as a practicing addict strips us of our spirituality. We lose our
connection with reality, giving more and more of ourselves to try to fill the emptiness within. Unfortunately,
we often don't discover that the addiction cannot deliver
what it promised until we've paid the high price of
spiritual atrophy.

We once made compulsive sexual behavior our Higher
Power, but it is only our real Higher Power who can
remove our obsessive attitudes and behaviors and can
make us sane. Seeking this Higher Power means changing directions completely. Step Two helps us find hope,
without which none of us can live. We come to this Step
as people emerging from a long, life-threatening journey through a wasteland. It is then, as beings of spirit
as well as of flesh, that we start another journey to a
Higher Power of light, joy, and unconditional love.

Step Two is a process, and I get all the time I need.

SK

A quiet conscience sleeps in thunder.
— *English proverb*

When our sexuality ruled our lives we lost our sense of right behavior and decency. We were so concerned with satisfying the demands of our addiction that we let our fantasies overrun our deepest convictions. Our morality and our values slipped away.

Even so, most of us eventually knew how far off the path we were, and we longed to find our way back to be at peace with ourselves. In the midst of our affliction, we began to hear a voice that told us we were not being true to ourselves. We were way off track and we knew it. We longed for the peace of a quiet conscience, but did not find it. We were alone and outside, in the cold.

That is why we came in to the warmth of a Twelve Step program. We need to return to our values and be at peace with ourselves. We can do it with the help of our friends in recovery and our Higher Power.

My conscience is a precious part of me, and I am learning to be truly in touch with it.

PW

Then comes the insight that All is God. One still realizes that the world is as it was, but it does not matter, it does not affect one's faith.
— Abraham Heschel

God is not an object to be possessed. As practicing addicts, we tried to possess people and change reality through sex. We needed the illusions of power and control to sustain us. There was no God except ourselves, and secretly we feared there was no one inside of us, only blackness, a void.

Step Three replaces the need to possess, the fear, and the void, with faith. When we turn our will and our lives over to the care of God as we understand God, we experience God. We let go of our self-will, no matter how haltingly, and trust that God will remake us according to spiritual principles.

Step Three deepens our commitment to recovery. We put willingness, openness, and honesty in our lives because we need them and because others have said they work. It's another act of faith. How do we find God? We don't. When we stop playing God and turn ourselves over to God, God finds us.

Thy will, not mine, be done.

SK

The main motive for "non-attachment" is a desire to escape from the pain of living, and above all from love, which, sexual or non-sexual, is hard work.

— George Orwell

In popular romances, love is often presented as a bed of roses — without the thorns. We may also have the idea that loving is always like falling in love — tricky, risky, thrilling, open-ended, a real high. And perhaps that is what we go on seeking when we act out in our addictive ways.

But love, over time, needs energy, loyalty, skill, patience, devotion — the same talents and dedication we need to bring to our work. Of course, love can be joyous and playful and childlike, but if it is to grow and mature it needs careful tending and hard work.

Love brings us into a close relationship with the pains as well as the joys of living. If we dare to become involved, intimate, committed, we will find ourselves on the way to becoming mature people in touch with the realities not of romance, but of life.

I know that loving means getting deeply involved with the joy and pain of living, and that's what I want.

PW

Do I contradict myself?
Very well, then, I contradict myself.
(I am large, I contain multitudes.)
                              — *Walt Whitman*

Step Four begins the process of restoring our relationship with ourselves. No matter how we structure an inventory, it inevitably reveals ourselves to us as we are. There is no bad news in our inventories, only the news of light and darkness together, in one person.

In the past we chose to see only what we wanted to see. It was necessary to be selective about what we believed we were because our addiction showed how we couldn't bear the truth. Now all that is behind us. Through a "searching and fearless moral inventory," we see that we are not bad, but human. With the help of our Higher Power and the sincere desire to be honest with ourselves, we face our character defects, especially fear, resentment, pride, and self-will. We also acknowledge our strengths, including our courage, willingness, and desire to change. The Fourth Step is our entrance into a wonderful new stage of growth.

Knowing myself is the first step to accepting and loving myself.

SK

Courage is like love; it must have hope for nourishment.

— *Napoleon*

Courage never operates in a vacuum; we are always courageous *about* something. And we need to believe that there will be some consequence to our acts of bravery. We are looking at the long term for some kind of salvation for ourselves and for others.

Love, too, needs a sense of future, time to develop and flower. Only passion lives for the moment, and passion, like the flame-red rose, often doesn't last out the year.

So love and courage are similar and often work together for our own good and the good of others. In our program we prize love and courage as we gain more wisdom and serenity. We come to believe in the long term and in things that endure. We know we can't change in a day, but with love and courage, and the hope on which they depend, we can do wonders.

I believe in my courage to change day by day.

PW

For nothing can be sole or whole
That has not been rent.

— *W. B. Yeats*

The power of Step Five is its ability to shatter our secrets. Once we share our inventory with another person, with the help and grace of our Higher Power, we acknowledge our membership in the human race. As our honesty strips away the charade of who we were, the dishonesty, isolation, fear, grandiosity, and self-will of our sex addiction receive a mortal blow.

It is healing to talk with another person. We simply can't accomplish the same thing by ourselves. Even though we may be afraid to share our inventory, with God's help we can trust the effort and let go of the outcome.

Every admission we make, and every secret we tell during our recovery will reflect who and where we are at that moment. Telling our secrets helps us give them up. Asking for help acknowledges our need for others and helps us let go of the past.

God, please help me find the humility and honesty to hold back nothing in my admitting to You, myself, and another person the exact nature of the harm I've caused myself and others.

SK

*The time to relax is when you don't have
time for it.*

— *Sydney J. Harris*

Many of us are workaholics, always pushing ourselves
to the limit, convincing ourselves that we are only happy
when we are working. We can't seem to find the time
for ourselves or for others as we rush though life. How
often we say, "I wish I could find the time to do this"
or "Why do I never have the time to see you these days?"

It is precisely when we are at our busiest and our
most frenzied that we need to set aside time for ourselves and for those we love. A child may need to be
with us; a loved one deserves intimacy. There is time
for these necessary things, and we will be enriched by
taking the time.

Those of us suffering from sex addiction are often
driven to keep busy in order to hide our feelings of
shame and unworthiness. As we get well, we will find
that we are setting more and more time aside for reflec-
tion and intimacy. These moments are precious markers
of our recovery.

I am learning to take time to be with myself and with others.

PW

Often the test of courage is not to die, but to live.
— *Vittorio Alfieri*

Step Six strengthens our relationship with God. Through it, we develop the willingness to let go of the character defects we admitted in Step Five. To be ready is to acknowledge that we cannot remove our own character defects. We tried that — it's called sex addiction. Instead, we turn with faith, trust, and humility to a Power greater than ourselves. We believe a Higher Power can and will remove our shortcomings.

We have often said we want to change. Step Six challenges us to act on what we say. If we want to live in recovery, we must be willing to give up our character defects. We must be willing to give up everything that keeps us from our Higher Power. We don't have to be perfectly willing, only as entirely willing as we can be at this moment. The point of readiness is the still center where we wait with confidence, knowing that our Higher Power is working in our lives.

Today, I will be open to the moments of readiness that come to me.

SK

It is easy to fly into a passion — anybody can do that — but to be angry with the right person to the right extent and at the right time and with the right object and in the right way — that is not easy, and it is not everyone who can do it.

— Aristotle

Perhaps we were brought up in a household where anger was taboo and voices were never raised. Perhaps everything was bottled up because we were afraid of anger. But we *were* angry.

It's hard to be angry appropriately. It needs to be learned, like so many things in our emotional life. If we haven't learned to direct our anger in appropriate ways, we may find ourselves flying into sudden, inexplicable, and unfocused rages that scare us and people around us. Or else we behave sullenly and irritably for no apparent reason. Or we get mad now for something that happened twenty years ago.

In our program we learn to direct our anger and get angry in a justifiable and appropriate way. It's good to get rid of our anger for the past so that we can concentrate on living fully in the present.

Today I'm going to try and deal honestly with my feelings, especially my anger.

PW

My creator, I am now willing that you should have all of me, good and bad. I pray that you now remove from me every single defect of character which stands in the way of my usefulness to you and my fellows. Grant me strength as I go out from here to do your bidding. Amen.
— Alcoholics Anonymous

When we reach the point where we ask God to remove our shortcomings, we are at the point of no return. When we ask God to remove our character defects, we let go completely. It is as if we were a beautiful statue waiting to be revealed from formless marble, and God is the sculptor. How exciting it is to be who we really are, free of the weaknesses that drove us as practicing sex addicts.

The humility we need to ask God to remove our shortcomings is taking an attitude of being teachable. As God chips away at our defects, we attain balance because the good qualities we possess can at last shine. We work Step Seven because we want to have more to give — to God, to ourselves, to others, and to life. Working Step Seven is an act of unconditional love on our part toward God and God's love toward us.

All I have to do is ask, humbly.

SK

There's nothing worse than taking something into your head: it turns into a revolving wheel that you can't control.

— Ugo Betti

When something really gets to us, it can easily become an obsession. We think of it morning, noon, and night, and worry about it like a dog guarding a bone.

Sex addicts are obsessed by fantasies that spin inside us like endless whirring wheels. In our affliction, we are unable to imagine real people in live situations. We keep repeating images that are real only in our fantasies. These fantasies close us off from a world of truth.

To break free, we need to take drastic action. We must reach out and talk to others and learn from their experiences. We must follow a path that leads outward into life and away from the spinning wheels of our obsessions. Thousands have worked the Steps and are now walking proudly on the open road of recovery. Let's join them.

I am learning to live a life away from my mad world of addiction and obsession. I am reaching out and getting free.

PW

I only ask to be free.

— Charles Dickens

Having had our relationship with God and with our-selves restored, we are finally ready to mend other rela-tionships. Making a list of people we have harmed and becoming willing to make amends to them begins the process of reconnecting us to other people so we can again feel part of humanity.

Many recovering people recommend that we include on our list our family, friends, creditors, and even those who have died. As sex addicts, we may also want to list those with whom we acted out, including former lovers. It is even possible to make a silent amend to someone we fantasized about being sexual with.

The crucial willingness to make amends comes when we allow ourselves our true feelings about how we hurt each person. Resentment, blame, grudges, and anger are not healing; taking responsibility for ourselves is. As ad-dicts we used other people in order to have our sub-stance: sex. It is this special soul-searing pain that Step Eight helps heal.

God, grant me the humility and honesty I need to make my list of people I have harmed and become willing to make amends to them all.

SK

Without forgiveness life is governed... by an
endless cycle of resentment and retaliation.
                              — *Roberto Assaglioli*

As recovering addicts we know the harm done to ourselves and others by our addiction. And yet, our illness may continue to be a breeding ground for resentment. Perhaps we think others are healthier and more successful than we are, and we imagine that they look down on us. We may imagine that other people have it in for us or are trying to harm us. While there may really be occasions when we truly have been wronged, most of our resentment is probably delusional.

Whatever the situation, it is clear that part of our recovery is forgiving ourselves and others, and making things right. Our program gives us the opportunity to identify, reveal, and turn over our defects of character. At a later stage, we prepare to make amends to those we have harmed by these defects.

In this way our program helps us break through the cycle of hurt and retaliation. We come to see that there is a way out of our addictive thinking; through forgiveness and acceptance, we can find serenity and peace.

I am following the Steps toward ending resentment and retaliation. I am learning to forgive and be forgiven.

*The A.A. program is one big amend broken
into twelve parts.*

— The Little Red Book

In Step Nine we go through the list of people we have
harmed and make amends to them one at a time. It is
never easy to go to someone and admit we've been
wrong. But although it's hard on the ego, it's good for
the self-esteem.

We know how deeply we long to leave the past behind
by our willingness to make amends. Whether God puts
someone in our path spontaneously or whether we plan
a letter or visit, our amends can be simple and from
the heart. Keeping in mind that we do not want to injure
anyone, we make our amends appropriate. For example,
many of us sex addicts may consider how honest we
want to be in revealing past sexual activity. Sometimes
such sincere words as, "I'm sorry I hurt you," are
enough. The right amend can also be a change in attitude or a change in behavior.

An amend is one of the most powerful ways we find
our way back. It is truly freeing.

*God will help me know the best amend for the situation.
I get all the time I need.*

SK

The most wasted day is that in which we have not laughed.

— *Chamfort*

When we are adrift in our sex addiction, we take ourselves very seriously and often lose contact with reality. We become lost in fantasy and obsession. Life becomes joyless because we can't see beyond our addiction, and we find no real satisfaction there. We lose touch with the joy and humor of life, and we find that everything around us and inside us is grim and dark.

One of the many positive signs of our return to health and sanity is our recovery of the gift of laughter. Each day as we gain more energy and zest for life, we move into the world and find many things that are humorous, in ourselves and in other people. We laugh, and find we are no longer alone.

Laughter is the mark of a healthy, happy human being. Laughter shows that we are truly a part of the human community. It is a sign that we are alive and on the way to recovery.

I am glad that I can laugh again and feel in touch with myself and others.

PW

*So live that you wouldn't be ashamed to sell
the family parrot to the town gossip.*
— *Will Rogers*

It is a challenge to live in the present, but Step Ten
gives us a way to do just that. It is a maintenance step,
a way to stay true to ourselves. As we continue to take
inventory of our attitudes and behavior, we find ourselves growing in self-acceptance and self-love. In the
past, the last thing we wanted to do was be honest. Now,
possessing serenity and faith, we can see that our shortcomings are only that: shortcomings. They are part of
who we are, and every part of ourselves is important.

Taking a personal inventory is not a way to sit in judgment of ourselves. Rather, it enables us to examine our
behavior with honesty and gentleness. It is an affirmation that growth is a process; we do it throughout our
lives. Taking time for a personal inventory is a way to
say that our needs are important, our good points are
important, and our character defects are important. We
are whole people, lovable just as we are.

*I will take time for an inventory today. I will admit my
wrongs, give myself credit for my accomplishments, and give
the day to God with gratitude.*

SK

August

There is nothing permanent except change.
— Heraclitus

Addiction convinced us that we could never change. We couldn't remember a time when we weren't lonely, isolated, shameful, hopeless. Our addiction had us convinced that we were unworthy and unlovable. We thought surely we must have been born that way.

In recovery we may not always be aware that we are changing, for change often takes place unnoticed and unfelt. It's like skiing or typing: there seem to be long periods when no improvement is noticeable, and then suddenly we make a breakthrough.

The law of life is change. Whether we realize it or not, we are always on the move, growing, developing. Our recovery may seem invisible at times, but it is happening. We are moving along the path, and each step means change and progress. Soon we will notice it and be glad.

I know I'm changing, and I see this as a joyful sign of my recovery from addiction.

PW

Love God, and do as you will.
— *St. Augustine*

Imagine yourself in a boat, far from land, dying of thirst. Little do you know that the water around you is fresh, not salty as you believe. All you have to do is reach down and drink it.

Step Eleven is our opportunity to drink as much of this fresh water as we want, whenever we want, because we live in the center of God's unimaginable grace and power. We know that we do not accomplish our own recoveries: God does. Our part is to be open to God's will, especially as we know it through prayer and meditation. The healing, restorative power of prayer and meditation starts the day right, ends it peacefully, and salvages it when it's falling apart. Through conscious contact with our Higher Power, we discover how to allow it to be the source of our energy. How this works is a mystery, and we can let it be so, grateful only for our ability to pray and God's willingness to respond. As the Big Book says, "Every day is a day when we must carry the vision of God's will into all of our activities."

In my Higher Power is true power: the power to be, the power to act, and the power to use both to recover.

SK

Better bend than break.

> — *Scottish proverb*

We may remember the story of the competition between the reed and the oak during a gale. As the wind howled, the oak boasted, while the reed said nothing. The wind became a tempest, and the reed bent down flexibly to the ground. The oak fell, uprooted.

Sometimes we seem strong but we are just being stubborn. We become rigid in our moral positions and don't even try to understand the problems of our children, friends, colleagues. We like to be thought of as uncompromising and tough.

Maybe we're frightened. Perhaps as addicts we fear that if we start to compromise we will be lost; one sign of weakness and the dam will burst and we'll be up to our old tricks again.

Let's not confuse rigidity with true strength. To be strong we need to be tolerant, responsive, and gentle. We need to be strong in a loving, flexible, human way. This is a central part of our recovery.

I will think about what it means to be strong in my mind and my heart.

FW

By this, the dreamer crosses to the other shore.
And by a like miracle, so will each whose work
is the difficult, dangerous task of self-discovery
and self-development be portered across the
ocean of life.

— *Joseph Campbell*

Step Twelve is the rousing affirmation that we have experienced the true miracle of a spiritual awakening and recovery. What a gift to be able to carry the message of recovery to those who still suffer from an addiction to sex. Through God's power, we are the channel of God's grace, giving ourselves unconditionally to life.

Each of us experiences recovery differently, and through our combined experience we find our voice, singly and as a fellowship. Somewhere there is someone who needs to hear that voice, feel the hope in our hearts, and see the peace in our eyes. There is no such thing as a good or bad recovery; there is only our recovery. It is priceless in our Higher Power's eyes, because in the end only our Higher Power knows what we went through to get where we are today. We come to this new life through Twelve simple Steps that we will never outgrow.

Now that I have surrendered myself to God, I praise and thank God through my life today.

SK

Anger as soon as fed is dead
'Tis starving makes it fat.
— Emily Dickinson

Many sex addicts have a problem with anger. We may have been sexually abused, neglected, or battered as children, and we may turn that abuse against ourselves or others in a vicious, repetitive cycle.

We need to talk about incidents that still torment us, and get angry at those who abused us. If we have been victimized, we are likely to go on being victims until we fight our way out of those early situations. Often, we can only do that by giving ourselves permission to vent anger as an affirmation of our self-worth, and not a contradiction of all we have been taught about being tolerant, forgiving, and peace-loving.

It is possible to hate the deed but to forgive the doer. We have the right to hate what happened to us, we have the right to be angry at people for their aggressive, hurt-ful acts, while being ready to forgive them as people who need love just as much as we do. If we keep our anger back, it will fester and come out in mean and petty ways. Let's not starve our anger, or it will rob us of our dignity and serenity.

I do have things to be angry about, and it is healthy for me to get angry at people when they abuse and humiliate me.

All loss is gain. Since I have become nearsighted,
I see no dust or squalor and, therefore, conceive
of myself as living in splendor.
— Alice James

Living in recovery can seem at times like coming full circle. We may be doing some of the same things we did as practicing addicts, but we're doing them now with different attitudes, a new enthusiasm and, best of all, gratitude.

In the painful days when we lived for the next sexual fix, all we could achieve was mere survival. A feeling of hopelessness and compulsivity pervaded every activity, even some of the ones we anticipated with delight.

Through our spiritual awakening, we can do the same things we did before, only much better. We can also take on responsibilities and challenges we never would have believed possible. The moment to stop and say a prayer of thanks is when we realize we've come full circle. We can also remember with gratitude the many recovering people who have freely shared their experience, strength, and hope so that we, too, might live.

I am part of the wonderful circle of life, of humanity, and of fellowship.

SK

The crow that mimics a cormorant gets drowned.

— *Japanese proverb*

When we are young we are vulnerable to the images of success that surround us — in sports, in politics, and in our social life. We watch our heroines and heroes perform, and we strive to emulate them. When the cormorant dives from a hundred feet, we'd love to follow.

As we get older, many of us don't manage to find out who we really are because we've been too busy trying to imitate others — in our dress, our way of talking, our business deals, our preferences, and our tastes. We often aped those who were considered "with it" at the time.

It's healthy to have role models, but they should reflect our true, emerging selves, and not be at the other end of the spectrum. As crows, we'd look silly diving from a hundred feet. Our challenge in recovery is to find out who we are and who we can be and go after that with all our energy. There's nothing wrong with being a crow.

I want to strive with all my heart to be myself.

PW

Miracles are instantaneous. They cannot be summoned, but come of themselves, usually at unlikely moments to those who least expect them

— Katherine Anne Porter

Nobody can force us to be in recovery or twist our arm to make us work our program. There might have been times when we wanted someone to, especially in the beginning, but those times pass. The longer we live in recovery, the more committed we become. We can be grateful that we've stayed with it, One Day at a Time. Through times of joy and sadness, through slips, tears, struggling with difficult problems, and during moments of peaceful fellowship with new friends, we can truly say that recovery is never boring.

Many of us came to the program because we had no place else to go. Through the mystery of our choices and God's grace, time goes by and we change. It is then we realize that the promises of recovery are coming true. As the Big Book states, the promises of recovery are being "fulfilled among us — sometimes quickly, sometimes slowly. They will always materialize if we work for them."

My gratitude and joy for the miracle of recovery are boundless.

SK

Art is meant to disturb.

— *Georges Braque*

Many great artists were neglected or even abused during their lifetime because their work was considered too provocative. Painters like Van Gogh, poets like Blake or Poe, and novelists like James Joyce were pushed out to the margins of society because their vision was too disturbing.

Most of us like a comfortable life, and those of us who are addicted to one high or another may not want to be troubled by new ways of seeing and imagining the world. Yet the day comes when our addiction no longer satisfies us and we long for a new vision and version of our lives. Art can help us in our recovery.

Art allows us to change our way of looking and living, even if at first the change is disturbing. Like artists, we can create new images and new patterns for our lives. At first, it may be painful. Old, comfortable habits die hard. But as we move forward step-by-step in our program, we come to see that it's exciting to be on the move and even at the frontier of new creative endeavors. Creativity, after all, comes from loving ourselves and others.

I can see that my new life will be full of the unknown, but that is what can make it exciting and creative.

God gave burdens, also shoulders.
                    — *Yiddish proverb*

Some days we wake up, and we know we can't get out of bed. We lie there, trying to force ourselves, but none of the usual motivations work. We may be depressed, we may be grieving, or we may simply be tired. It's hard to resist the temptation to believe that everyone else is functioning with ease. "They all show up for work. What's wrong with me?" The more frantic we become, the more likely we may lapse into old ways of thinking and behaving in order to get moving.

If we feel we can't get out of bed, there's usually a good reason why. We can give ourselves permission to discover it. By being honest, we will discover how to take care of ourselves. Maybe it's a day to stop and nurture ourselves, not force ourselves to keep going. Only we know what we really need. We do not have to compare ourselves to others or apologize for what we are going through. Instead, we can be gentle, giving our bodies, emotions, and spirits what they require. We can turn the day over to God's will.

I pray for the willingness to make this a day of healing. I will be part of my own renewal.

SK

It is a luxury to be understood.
— *Ralph Waldo Emerson*

Many sex addicts feel that, from their earliest days, they have been misunderstood. Perhaps we went to a parent for comfort and were sexually abused; perhaps we spoke of our need for affection and were exploited by a brother or sister or by a friend. Our messages and calls for human contact were grossly misinterpreted. We wanted affection, but we got abuse.

What a relief to be working and talking in a group where others genuinely respond to us! We know now that even our darkest thoughts can be shared and our basest actions are understood. There is nothing we cannot say to the group because it has become a place of trust and responsiveness.

As we learn to express ourselves knowing that we will be heard and accepted, we feel stronger and more integrated into the human community. We are learning to talk our way out of our loneliness and our sickness.

I know I am beginning to trust others because they listen to me and give me understanding.

PW

Everyone suddenly burst out singing.
— *Siegfried Sassoon*

The child within us wants to come out and play. The adult in us may resist, but why not do it anyway? Having fun, being playful, and letting go of rigid personas is as necessary to recovery as good food and loving relationships.

Having fun is an attitude as well as an activity. We can have a good time with everything we do — well, almost everything. But dancing around the living room, taking a day off work, doing something artistic, taking a child to the zoo — the world is full of things that are enjoyable. It might even be fun to make a list of things that are fun.

Being willing to have fun frees the spontaneous, goofy, carefree parts of ourselves. We can show that side to people and practice not caring what they think. While we don't have to abandon our boundaries, it's good to take a risk and let go. In the end it's our spirits that are freed. Who knows? We might even jump off the high pinnacle of the adult world and laugh as we take the fall.

Discovering what I have fun at, and doing it, helps me grow in my recovery.

SK

Fate is non-awareness.

— *Jan Kott*

We tend to blame fate for things that happen to us. Some of us go around looking at life saying, "If only. . ." Bad luck, other people, our childhood — everything outside or beyond us is to blame in this version of our "fate." If only. . .

It would be well to look inside ourselves when we feel the urge to think this way. We need insight and self-awareness. If we follow our thoughts and emotions honestly, frankly, and fearlessly, we will often find we have been blind to many things that come from within ourselves. We, not fate, were responsible.

Awareness comes with honesty and is a vital part of recovery. Being more aware, we learn to situate ourselves more solidly in our own history and take responsibility when the responsibility is ours.

I can stop turning against life and blaming people and events for my own shortcomings.

FW

The reduction of the universe to a single being, the expansion of a single being even to God, this is love.

— *Victor Hugo*

There is a profound connection between sexuality and spirituality. Both are expressions of the deepest parts of who we are; both touch our core being. Many of the qualities we associate with spirituality may be experienced when we are sexual: transcendence, self-forgetfulness, ecstasy, union with another, integration of all of oneself.

There is nothing to fear in exploring all the dimensions of sexuality: emotional, mental, physical, and, especially, spiritual. In the past we cut off our spiritual selves in order to be sexual. Now we no longer have to pay that price or suffer that deep disconnection. We can bring all of ourselves, including our spirituality, into our sexual expression. Both come from our Higher Power. As our recovery progresses, we will know at a deeper and deeper level that our sexuality is nothing to fear or avoid. The addiction cannot harm us when God is present and our bodies and spirits are united.

God, I trust you to guide me in the healthiest and highest expressions of my sexuality.

SK

A new broom is good for three days.
— Italian proverb

We like to think that a new broom sweeps clean — once and for all. We zip through our program, and that's it. No more worries. No more acting out. Home free!

One of the reasons we introduce ourselves as sex addicts at our meetings is that we realize our illness will continue to be a part of who we are. Many of us can hardly remember a time before recovery when we weren't addicted to sexual fantasies and acting out. This doesn't mean we're nothing but sex addicts — obviously we all lead varied lives and have unique personalities. But we are all subjected to the driving force of our obsessions and compulsions.

We need to be equally persistent in our program. It's no good dropping into meetings once every two months and treating our program like a club. We need to be tough, resolute, vigilant, and unfailingly honest if we are to get out from the shadow and shame of our addiction. And we need to be constantly coming back to the program for more help and support.

I know I need to be faithful to my program and vigilant with respect to my addiction.

PW

Envy is more implacable than hatred.
— *de La Rochefoucauld*

Many of us, at times, have felt envious of other people. We envy those who have what we want: more money, more self-confidence, a happy relationship, a more interesting life. In the past, we defined our desires according to our addictive values, and the addiction told us we needed more, always more.

If we look beneath our envy, what will we find? Sadness? Anger? Feelings of deprivation? These are real emotions, reflecting childhoods and present lives spent struggling with loss. No wonder we lapse into envy; it's painful to face the magnitude of the losses we've endured and the needs that have gone unmet.

One way to get beyond envy is to work toward healing the past by filling up the present. We can recognize that envy is corrosive and disrespectful. It turns the people we envy into objects and separates us from them. Our peace of mind comes from living in the present and being comfortable with who we are. We can't live someone else's life, only our own.

If I feel envious today, I will gently bring myself back into the present by realizing how worthwhile I am and how richly I am blessed.

SK

The old woman I am going to become is quite
different from the woman I am now.
— *George Sand*

One thing that really scares sex addicts is the feeling
that we may go on and on living the same scenarios
until we die. No change, no freedom, no love, just
the mechanical routine of our obsessive thinking and
acting out.

Let's protest vehemently against this version of our
lives. We have so many possibilities, so many directions
to pursue. We see others in our groups change and
reach upward and grow. We have time and energy
and purpose, so what's holding us back?

The ball and chain of our addiction kept us limping
along the road, but we can now break the chain and
find a new way to walk and a new path to follow. In
our hearts we know we can do it, if we are patient and
gentle with ourselves and consistent and brave with
our decisions.

The time to begin to change is now.

I don't want to keep hesitating and waiting; I know I am
changing and I want to continue to grow.

PW

*Therefore, will I trust you always, though I may
seem to be lost and in the shadow of death.
I will not fear, for you are ever with me, and
you will never leave me to face my perils alone.*
— Thomas Merton

Many of us have felt at times that we don't know where
we're going. Maybe we've just made an important change,
like leaving a job or a relationship. Perhaps we feel far
away from our Higher Power and don't know how to
find our way back. Or we might be entering a new stage
of recovery, which often entails a deeper commitment
to our recovery program and insecurity about the future.

During the times we have no answers, it may be
enough simply to ask the questions. Our inclination as
sex addicts is to be in control, to put our minds to work
and figure things out. But some things simply can't be
dealt with only with logic. All we can do is ask the questions, have faith in the answers as our Higher Power
reveals them to us, and let go.

We find new faith by working through those situations where we don't have the answer right away. Part
of life's wonder is its mystery. It takes faith to not only
accept the mystery, but to embrace and love it.

*Life is a question mark. Today is a day to accept and cherish
that in my life.*

SK

Thanks to art, instead of seeing one world (our own), we see it multiplied.

— Marcel Proust

In our active addiction we tended to have a single, narrow view of ourselves and the world. We thought that everyone was obsessed by fantasies and erotic images; we saw others as mere doubles of ourselves.

One of the great joys of reading is to enter other people's lives. We often come to know fictional characters even better than our friends because a novelist can give us the illusion of being all-powerful and all-knowing. So we get a special "inside view," and many people in books become familiar and dear to us.

Reading can take us out of ourselves and expand our views of other people. We learn that, indeed, "it takes all sorts to make a world," and our lives become less isolated through contact with others. The power of art is to deepen and enrich this perception of ourselves in relationship to the world. Through reading, watching plays and films, or exploring a painter's world, we learn how varied and fascinating other people are.

I am glad I can get to know other people's lives by becoming involved in their artistic expressions and by talking to others about what I read and see.

PW

What we don't know supports what we do know.

— *Bill Moyers*

One way we show respect for ourselves and others is by respecting whatever life brings us. What prevented that in the past was our preoccupation with sex and with having our own way. Now, we live our lives on a different rhythm: one of letting go. It is that rhythm to which we must pay attention.

At times letting go feels like doing nothing, and doing nothing feels like standing still. But letting go is not the same as standing still. It is active, not passive. Letting go focuses our attention on life in the present, living it fully moment by moment, rather than in a fantasy future that seems to promise the outcome we crave.

It has been said that the light of God's love is so bright that it appears as darkness to us. When we feel we're living in darkness, we may be living in the all-encompassing light of God's love and compassion for our struggle. We can trust the daily evidence of that love and know we are safe.

My struggles have dignity because I face them with faith in my Higher Power.

SK

Failures are usually the most conceited of men.
— *D. H. Lawrence*

If we believe deep down that we are worthless, we may feel we have to cover up our failures. Sometimes we do this by becoming boastful and grandiose in our attitude toward ourselves and others. We protect ourselves by putting on airs.

Other people may be taken in for a while. But sooner or later, our real feelings about ourselves will begin to show through, like an old painting that has been imperfectly covered over. Eventually we may begin to refuse positions of responsibility or "flunk out" of relationships. We can get to the point where we dare not take risks, for we know we will fail. Our sexual addiction makes us lose touch with our real selves.

When we begin to find and create ourselves anew, we will become more humble and more modest in our dealings with others. Now that we are getting well, we don't need to keep others at a distance through conceited behavior.

I don't need to pretend to be someone else now that I am becoming content with myself.

FW

*Can such thing be, And overcome us like a
summer's cloud, Without our special wonder?*
— *William Shakespeare*

When our ability to participate again in life is restored
through recovery, we also rediscover the gift of commitment. Maybe the commitment is to raising a child,
doing a job we love, earning a degree, or working on
a special relationship. It is a moment of wonder when
we have something in our lives that requires the best
we have to give.

During times of doubt or struggle, we may question
what we've gotten ourselves into. But an activity or a
person to which we give ourselves wholly and freely
is evidence of our Higher Power in our lives. If the
commitment is to something God has asked us to do,
we can know absolutely that God will help us take care
of it. The time we need will come, money will come,
support will come, and the energy and enthusiasm we
need will come. Although it may appear that things are
simply going our way, we can trust God is giving them
to us so our task can be accomplished.

*Today offers me a wonderful opportunity to fulfill my commit-
ments in peace and grace. I am being looked after.*

SK

*He was so benevolent, so merciful a man that
he would have held an umbrella over a duck
in a shower of rain.*

— Douglas Jerrold

We are often in too much of a hurry to pause and
be attentive to the simple needs of others — an elderly
person crossing the road, a man having trouble with
his car, a child looking for a sign of love.

It seems that in a period when so many of us have
plenty of leisure, we end up with so little time. We've
all been through periods when we're so busy producing
and consuming that we don't take the time to share our
ideas and our feelings, or to show compassion. But there
are plenty of people crying out for care and affection,
people who are sick, who can't read, who simply need
a kind word and a helping hand.

We can resolve to care more, share more, and be more
attentive to the desires and needs of others. Benevo-
lence and mercy can be natural outcomes of our commitment to "practice these principles in all our affairs."

---

*I am a fortunate person and I want to share my talents and
good fortune with others.*

PW

Tis heaven alone that is given away,
Tis only God may be had for the asking.
— *James Russell Lowell*

Our relationship with our Higher Power is like any other relationship — it changes and deepens with time, and it requires effort. That's why the word conscious — in terms of conscious contact — is important in seeking to improve our relationship with a Higher Power. It takes a sense of consciousness to have a relationship with God. To be conscious is to be aware, to be in touch with reality, to live in the present. It is to have a sense of who we are, a sense of how we are different from everyone else.

It is this sense of personal uniqueness that our Higher Power invites us to bring to our relationship. As recovering sex addicts, we seek to experience greater conscious contact with God because to do so is to be more alive, spiritually, and in other ways. The more alive we feel, the easier it is to surrender our will to God's will. Surrendering takes trust, and trust in our Higher Power is difficult when we don't feel part of life. Carrying out God's will is only possible when we trust ourselves and the God within us who empowers us to live fully each day.

May I be open today to greater conscious contact with my Higher Power, seeking only to know and do God's will.

SK

No objects of value. . .are worth risking the
priceless experience of waking up one more day.
— Jack Smith

Every now and then, it's a good thing to strip life down to the essentials, the bare necessities. Close up the house, go off on a sailing trip, change careers, take a risk — we all need to occasionally face the world anew and get a fresh start.

We don't necessarily have to take extreme measures or act impulsively to realize the validity, the importance of being in touch with the simple things in life. But if we're too involved with toys, luxuries, and busy lifestyles, we buffer ourselves against reality and exist rather than live.

Daybreak, bird song, clouds flying, a favorite photograph, a well-loved quotation, the taste of waffles, wood smoke, starlight — these can give texture and genuine thrill to our lives. We need the wonder and joy that come with a simple, healthy life.

I'm tired of turmoil and clutter; I can keep a clearer vision with the simple things in life.

PW

There is no greater enemy to those who would please than expectation.

— *Montaigne*

Does this sound familiar: "Why did she do it like that? That's not the way I would have done it." How about this: "I don't understand why he's acting that way. What's wrong with him?" When we start to say things like this, we can stop and look inside ourselves. Chances are, we'll find expectations. When we want people to act and live according to our wishes, we have set ourselves up as arbiters of their behavior. Somewhere within ourselves, we cling to the idea that we know the best way.

Underneath our expectations may lurk such feelings as fear, insecurity, grandiosity, or anger. We worry that we can't control what's happening — and we're right, we can't. But the more we respect other people's right to make their own mistakes, to express their uniqueness, and to grow in their own time, the more freedom we have to do the same. We can use our power for our own good, rather than give it away to hidden or not-so-hidden expectations.

Am I setting myself up for disappointment by my expectations, or am I realistic about what I am expecting from myself, other people, and life?

SK

Power is the ultimate aphrodisiac.
— *Henry Kissinger*

As a result of our addiction, many of us lost our sense of power. We had to admit we were powerless to control our sexuality; it had been controlling us. Working the First Step is a move away from a battleground on which we were always the losers.

In our groups and in our program we learn to speak about a Higher Power — a spirit or a force that is not ours to deploy but that transcends us. By surrendering our egos to this new Power, we get back in touch with our place in the scheme of things and discover the spiritual direction and pattern of our lives.

Of course, there will always be those, in government and elsewhere, for whom power rather than love is the main driving force in life. But what do we mean by "power" and how does it satisfy us? As addicts we tried to use power against our addiction, but the result was always defeat. Finally, we found what many before us have found: the only true, abiding power is the power of love.

In my recovery I am learning to redefine power and see its relationship with love.

PW

A soft answer turneth away wrath.
— *Prov. 15:1*

One of the most important things we learn in recovery is to be gentle with ourselves. Why is gentleness particularly important for a recovering sex addict? Our common experience has taught us that sex addiction can be violent. Whether we've been in a violent relationship, contemplated suicide, or been violent in other ways, sex addiction has shown how it can batter and harden us. It demeans every effort we make to feel good about ourselves.

The wisdom of recovery helps us learn how to be kind to ourselves and others. In our groups, we treat each other with compassion, knowing that gentle attitudes and behavior heal the addiction's harshness and violence. To be gentle does not mean avoiding pain or being dishonest. Rather, it helps us be strong in a way that does not damage us, but restores us. Gentleness gives us room to breathe. It creates a safe place within, so we can learn to love ourselves again.

I will be gentle with myself today.

SK

Wisely and slow. They stumble that run fast.
— Shakespeare

There are many sayings and proverbs that advise us to take our time. This popular wisdom, often coming from people far from hectic cities, speaks of life's natural rhythm and tempo. It reminds us that we are better off if we stay in touch with the measured turning of the world reflected in the passing of the seasons.

Many of us may have forgotten to take time to look at the stars or watch a bird in flight. It's as if we have our eyes always on success and our noses to the grindstone. And from there, how easy it is to move back into actively practicing our addiction and to end up blotting out the real world altogether.

Time is given to us all, to measure and lend form to our roles as participants in creation. Let's take time to enjoy it. We can find more than mere relaxation in time; we may even discover wisdom.

I can slow down to experience the rhythm of time in the here and now.

PW

Thy love is strong; thy faithfulness, everlasting.
— Ps. 100:5

Many of us thought when we were acting out that we wanted sex. But it wasn't sex we really wanted; it was love. The needs that drove us are a part of all loving relationships — acceptance, validation, attention, touching — but we experienced them as a hunger for sex. We had sex and love all mixed up.

To sort such things out alone is too much for us, but we can use the Twelve Step program, our sisters and brothers in recovery, and our Higher Power. Many of us have found our first experience of unconditional love through our Higher Power's love.

In recovery, we learn that we cannot control love. To love is to let go. We also cannot control the people who love us; their love is a gift. Once we accept our need for love and give up trying to meet the need alone, we can free ourselves from the illusion that being sexual will bring us love. We can concentrate on the real love that exists in our lives. We can feel it, nurture it, sustain it, and, finally, give it.

The love within me is infinite. To express it in whatever I do is to express my unique spirit.

SK

Courage is grace under pressure.
                    — *Ernest Hemingway*

Sexual addiction was a force that constantly caused us to act in demeaning and degrading ways. We went out to buy something for a friend and found ourselves acting out; we did errands to help our family and spent all our money on pornography or visits to prostitutes. We lived under the powerful pressure of our affliction and gradually became emotionally bankrupt.

Is there hope for us? Yes, as we listen to the Serenity Prayer and find in ourselves the courage to change the things we know we can change. We can learn to behave differently, with the help of the group, the Twelve Step program, and our Higher Power.

In listening to others, in sharing their struggles, in trusting in life and our place in the universe, we will come to find the courage to choose to turn our lives proudly toward the new with hope.

I know I am gaining the courage to turn toward a new life. This new life will help me resist the pressure of my addiction.

PW

September

Even the cry from the depths is an affirma-
tion: Why cry if there is no hint of hope of
hearing?

— *Martin Marty*

What happens to a girl who doesn't get the help she needs from her parents? What becomes of a boy who reaches out, time and again, to parents who don't respond to his needs? What kind of life awaits the victim of childhood sexual abuse who has no one to turn to for help?

We know some of the answers to those questions because, for many of us, our childhoods included suffering alone, in silence. Help was asked for, but never received. Trust was betrayed when we reached out.

We can't condemn ourselves if we have a hard time asking for help. Healing is a process; trusting is a process; risking is a process. We can reach out only as much as we are able to this moment. We must trust that through our recovery, over time, our sense of dignity and clarity will be reestablished. Day by day we will find ourselves better able to ask for what we need.

My wounds from the past do not have to be fully healed in order for me to start anew.

SK

No one can make you feel inferior without your consent.

— *Eleanor Roosevelt*

Even though we deny it, we still may secretly want to be hurt by others, since, in some obscure way, we think we deserve it. As addicts we had lost our good opinion of ourselves; we often indulged in actions that placed us in situations of humiliation and debasement. It is a sad truth that sex addicts can feel comfortable there, and find release from tension in degrading acts.

Let's resolve to reject humiliation. We are learning, by talking with others, that life is rich and varied and open — and we want to join in. We do not have to continue to find false comfort and release in acts that come back to haunt and humiliate us.

There is no more room in our lives for feelings of inferiority and worthlessness. Our program helps us gain self-esteem and a sense of the true value of our lives.

I don't wish to be humiliated by situations and by other people. I deserve to do what makes me feel good about myself.

PW

*When you realize there is nothing lacking, the
whole world belongs to you.*
                                      — *Tao Te Ching*

Working the Twelve Steps is the process of being
and becoming. It is finding, knowing, and accepting who
we are. It is having the willingness to fall down,
stumble around, and make mistakes. It is being in tune
with the constant process of death and rebirth that is
part of life's rhythm.

Each of us has an internal timetable — the rhythm
of our spirit. Discovering what it is and living according
to its direction can bring us untold serenity and joy.
It also brings us energy, because we're not fighting ourselves and reality. So often, we are our own worst enemy.
But to face who we are and to learn from it is to be
created anew. In the process, we discover our own
truths. Maybe that's part of what a spiritual awakening
is; seeing the truth in a new way.

Living according to the guidance of our spirit and in
harmony with our body, mind, and emotions is a solitary journey, but one that brings us close to other people
and to life. It takes patience, and it brings true peace.

---

*I am able to trust that in my recovery I am learning new
things as I need to learn them. I am comfortable with the
pace of my recovery.*

SK

*If you look at life one way, there is always cause
for alarm.*

— *Elizabeth Bowen*

A narrow view, especially one that is attached to an obsession, is going to give us a very partial perspective on life. As sex addicts, we may come to believe that everyone is always fantasizing, acting out, getting involved in some kind of sexual escapade, and being miserable. That's the way the world is, from one point of view. And it's scary.

In our program we learn to reach out to others. As we do so, we see things differently, as if we put a different lens on our camera. We get a new perspective. We become involved, caring, committed. We didn't know life could be so rich and give so much. Now we see others as well as ourselves.

What made the difference? Sanity. When we stopped seeing things only from our crazy, addicted point of view, we returned to sobriety and love and sane behavior. We learn to look at things in new ways as we practice the Steps and ask for the help of our Higher Power.

I feel joyful now that I see the world with new eyes.

PW

*Perhaps the most important thing we can under-
take toward the reduction of fear is to make
it easier for people to accept themselves; to like
themselves.*

— *Bonaro Overstreet*

We may be going about our lives when, suddenly, we
become aware that we're feeling anxious or uncomfortable
or insecure. But what we're feeling, underneath, is afraid.
Even when we're not conscious of it, fear can drain our
concentration and deplete our confidence.

Everyone feels afraid; it is a part, even an affirmation of
being human. Fear can be a healthy, energizing response
in some situations — such as when we take a risk or
strike out in a new direction.

When we're fearful, it can be reassuring to remember
that, in the end, success or failure aren't what's important.
If, in any situation, we do the best we can and learn from
our experiences, then we've nothing to fear. Still, when
we're feeling fear, it's important to know that the people
who love us will go on loving us. Sometimes, we may
just need to hear someone say, "I know you can do it;
I have faith in you." Then, fearful or not, we move forward,
our fear balanced by faith and our willingness to try.

---

*God, please take away my fear or help me bear it, if that's
what I must do. I am always in Your care.*

SK

If you hate a person, you hate something in him that is part of yourself.
— *Hermann Hesse*

Hatred, like anger, corrodes and eats away at us, and we often end up being the losers. Our lives can be wrecked by the resentments and hostilities we feel for others.

Why? Because hatred paralyzes us and prevents us from moving forward. How often, as practicing addicts, did we become fixed in ugly feuds and rivalries, unable to get on with our lives?

As we become clear-sighted about our hatreds we find that they are often really directed at parts of ourselves that we dislike or even fear. We may hate noise because we were afraid of it as children; we may detest others' sexual preferences because we fear they may secretly be ours.

By being honest with ourselves we can get at the root of our anger and hatred. Then we can deal with these feelings and let them be carried away by the winds of time.

As I meditate I realize that my anger and hatred is often directed at myself. Now I am ready to work to get free of the hatred that cripples me.

PW

You gain strength, courage, and confidence by every experience in which you really stop to look fear in the face. You are able to say to yourself, "I lived through this horror. I can take the next thing that comes along."
— Eleanor Roosevelt

One of the miracles of recovery from sex addiction is that it gives us courage in the face of life's darker realities. We can help others face addiction, depression, or illness because we've been there too. We've gone through so much, and we've come out the other side. We understand the fear.

What a tremendous gift that can be to others, especially for those who come into recovery after us. Our presence, our support, our unconditional love, and our nonjudgmental attitude are often just what another suffering addict needs. Our experiences as practicing sex addicts have given us understanding and wisdom. We have the perspective to be practical and realistic when necessary. We have the empathy to be compassionate. We have the strength and clarity to keep our boundaries in the face of another's addiction. Our courage is our recovery in action, and for that we can be grateful.

I go through difficulties so that I can be helped, and so that I can later help someone else.

SK

No legacy is so rich as honesty.
— *Shakespeare*

As sex addicts, we've spent much of our lives living a lie. We were split into two people, Dr. Jekyll and Mr. Hyde, and one of the two could never speak out, tell the truth, own up. Mr. Hyde gradually took over until everything was fraud, deception, and betrayal. And then we came to see a life in ruins.

Beginning recovery meant finding ways for these two sides of ourselves to work together. We knew we needed to find a way to win the trust and confidence of both Dr. Jekyll and Mr. Hyde before one tore the other to pieces.

There is one way in: honesty. Mr. Hyde works only in the darkness of deceit and opens up to the light that streams in when we speak openly and honestly. And this light endures: honesty doesn't only give us momentary insight; it leaves a legacy that lasts a lifetime.

However hard it is, I am resolved to be open and honest with myself as I work my program.

PW

Solitude: A good place to visit, but a poor place to stay.

— *Josh Billings*

One trait shared by sex addicts is that we don't like to ask for help. We often sit in our Twelve Step meetings telling each other how hard it is to ask for help, and it sometimes seems we spend a lot of energy talking about it, but not asking for help.

Since many of us grew up with messages of isolation and shame being constantly reinforced, help can seem like a luxury reserved for other people. We think we don't deserve it. We think we should be able to handle everything. We fail to realize we need help because we're used to living in crisis. We tell ourselves our concerns and problems aren't important enough to bother people with. Then, when life gets complicated, we blame ourselves for feeling overwhelmed and unable to act.

But we do deserve help. We deserve all the help we want and need, whether it's a ride home when our car won't start or a friend's arms to hold us when we're crying. We're worth the time, effort, and concern of others not because we're different, but because we're the same.

Today, I will take the risk of asking for help, if help is what I need.

SK

A hard beginning makes a good ending.
— *John Heywood*

The First Step of our program was the hardest for many of us. We had to admit that the lives we had gotten used to — *our lives* — had become unmanageable. We could no longer continue to function in our addiction where we were mere pawns in a game we always lost. But for some of us, that life was the only one we knew, and we had to learn to change it and change it at the root. That was tough, and we knew it would be.

But our program offers a new way of relating to ourselves and others. We don't have to continue to go it alone. In the old system, the addiction system, we were always alone and that is why we always lost. In recovery, we are part of a group in which we can learn to feel a sense of belonging and shared affection. We no longer feel alone and powerless, but proud members of a new community.

The First Step is hard, yet we do have support and love from others, and our program opens the door to a new life.

I am not afraid to take the First Step because I know it is leading me into new ways of achieving health, sanity, and love.

PW

Without discipline, there's no life at all.
— *Katharine Hepburn*

We all have deadlines we must meet. We have bills to pay, responsibilities at work, children with school projects — all the innumerable small markers that push life forward.

When we realize we're procrastinating, we need to be committed to not shaming ourselves. Procrastination is not an indication that we have failed. How realistic would it be if we looked forward to doing unpleasant things? It's human to avoid what we'd rather not do.

As we free ourselves from the burden of perfectionism, we're free to better accept our responsibilities. Meeting deadlines as well as we can, one at a time, pays off in serenity and a manageable life. When we are crisis-ridden, we are forced to live by other peoples' demands, rather than by our choices. In the face of procrastination, resentment, or perfectionism, we can turn to Step Ten for an inventory. We can forgive ourselves, try to laugh at ourselves, live in the present, and keep going. Today can be better than yesterday.

I may as well admit it — there's probably something I'm avoiding. Is today the day to do it?

SK

The great law of culture: let each become what he is capable of becoming.
— *Thomas Carlyle*

Each of us is unique, precious, human. We need to join in the movements of life and culture that encourage us to grow and change and live out the fullness of our potential.

By remaining immersed in our addiction, we are joining the dead in life, those who deny the possibility of growth and becoming. Addiction is a stunting illness that holds back the healthy forward movement of life.

In our recovery there are moments of hesitation and even of relapse. When this happens we do not lose faith in ourselves because we are constantly strengthened by working our program. We gain insight by following the Steps, and we find support and strength in our groups and our Higher Power. And so we continue to reconnect with our own rhythm and pattern of growth.

I am part of a living culture and capable of change and growth.

PW

Friendship is a strong and habitual inclina-
tion in two persons to promote the good and
happiness of one another.
                              — *Eustace Budgell*

A woman in the program passed on one of her most important beliefs about relationships. It's this: "The person with the greater need comes first. This means there are times I will consciously choose to set aside my own needs, feelings, or concerns because someone else's need is greater. If I visit a friend in the hospital, it isn't the time to go on and on about how I've accepted a new job and am moving across the country."

We know that the more we progress in recovery, the more we'll develop relationships to turn to for support. And, of course, we have the best resource of all — ourselves. Our ability to guide, support, and nurture ourselves increases without our even being aware of it. The self-centeredness and selfishness we possessed as practicing sex addicts begins to disappear. We don't always have to vie for attention or have our own way. We can decide to put someone else first, not out of martyrdom, but out of respect and love.

When in doubt, I will remember: The one with the greater need comes first.

SK

Nothing will content him who is not content with little.

— *Greek proverb*

Our addiction gives us grandiose fantasies but not much satisfaction. We think we need to own a ton of stuff and spend a bundle to be happy. We often talk as if we have a big vision, but we don't notice what is in front of us. We can spend our lives missing what is really there.

We may notice on a camping trip how good it is to be surrounded only by the bare necessities — an open fire, a pot of stew, one knife, one fork, one spoon, a sleeping bag, and some basic protection against the cold, wind, and rain. We aren't spending time moving things around, needing things, buying things, moving things again, taking things back. At times like that we relax and really open our eyes to see.

Wisdom can mean taking delight in simple things; when we do this, we are never bored or boring.

I'm going to take time out to enjoy the simple things of life.

PW

Extremists think "communication" means agreeing with them.

— *Leo Rosten*

A woman was talking to a woman friend about her difficulties with a male colleague at work. When she finished, her friend said, "It's hard, isn't it, when someone else doesn't speak our language?"

So often men and women aren't speaking the same language. Someone who cries at work runs the risk of being called overemotional, or someone who sticks to the task at hand, no matter what, is perceived as cold and insensitive.

As practicing addicts, we relied on sex to define our behavior and our roles. We thought sex was always the highest form of expression and communication. Now we are trying to find new ways to communicate, especially nonsexual ways. The solution is not to speak the same language to the point of eradicating our masculinity or femininity when we deal with the opposite sex. Rather, we can look for a common language that still affirms our uniqueness as human beings.

My style of communication — how I express myself — is always evolving. I will let myself be who I am.

SK

Beware lest you lose the substance by grasping
at the shadow.

— *Aesop*

When we are addicted to sex, we grasp only at the shadow of things. We neither relate to people as if they are real, nor do we communicate as mature, loving people. Instead, we pursue phantoms, and, in the end, we find only dissatisfaction.

Sex addiction diminishes and demeans us as much as it allows us to see things only as extensions of ourselves. We become afraid of individuality and differences. We allow ourselves to see other people only as reflections of ourselves.

In recovery, we've come to need substance in our lives. It's when we work at real problems and connect with people as they are that we feel truly alive. For a good relationship to grow, we need to give and receive genuine affection.

In our groups we find substance and particularity. We find authentic people who are learning not to be afraid to extend themselves and who come to meet and greet us. We learn to live and love as vital, whole people in the real world.

I am learning to get out of the shadows and darkness of my addiction and live in a world of substance, reality, and love.   FW

*Now, let the weeping cease; let no one mourn
again. For the love of God will bring you peace.
There is no end.*

— *Sophocles*

When we look back on our life, we may feel again
the pain of how things used to be. But we know that
our life doesn't ever have to be as difficult as it once
was. It never has to be as out of control, as unmanageable, as terrifying. It isn't necessary for our sex addiction
to haunt us at every turn. Time has moved on, as it must.
The past is over and we've begun to know real safety.

Maybe we would have to abandon the program and
our commitment to recovery for quite some time before
we went back completely to how we acted and lived
as practicing sex addicts. We may slip today or some
day in the future; there are no promises of perfection.
We can never forget that we're sex addicts and only a
decision away from acting out. But that's different from
going back to the beginning, before our new life. Each
day we choose not to leave recovery strengthens our
heart so that we no longer want to go back.

*I will live One Day at a Time. I trust that I have all the
time I need.*

SK

*They are ill discoverers that think there is no
land, when they see nothing but sea.*
— Francis Bacon

When we are lost at sea, we may think that there is
no such thing as land, so immense and frightening is
the ocean that surrounds us. Nothing but huge stretches
of grey, heaving water and the fear that we aren't going
to make it. We cringe and withdraw from rational
thought and action. We become sick at heart.

So it is with our addiction. At times it seems that our
sex addiction is all we have, all we are. As long as we
can remember and as far as we can see into the future,
that's all there is.

We must shake ourselves free of that kind of obsessive thinking. We know there is land ahead and help
at hand. We have seen other people recover and we have
known recovery ourselves. There have been whole
days, weeks, months, when we haven't been lost in
the sea of our addiction. Our program and our sisters
and brothers are our lifeline. We will make a safe pas-
sage home if we believe in ourselves and our program.

---

*I am learning to think in a rational manner about myself
and my addiction. I know I will return to sanity if I continue to have faith in myself and my program.*

We yield, and we realize God has wrought something in us, and that the wings of our souls have learned to beat the upper air.

— *Anonymous*

Where are our resting places? Where are the free spaces where we find nurturing and peace? For some of us, it is within ourselves: a place where we live quietly, engaged in inarticulate creation. We go to that silent space because we are safe there. We find what we need to be replenished until we are ready to go into the world again.

For some of us, the resting places are primarily outside ourselves: the earth, the sea, the mountains. We call this "getting away from it all," but it's really going to something we need as much as we need air and food. We all will find a resting place in anything to which our hearts call us: music, a journal, books on recovery, solitude. We all need sanctuary; time to be recreated; time to become reconnected to who we truly are.

I will praise You, my God, for, within my solitary sanctuary, You are always with me.

SK

Art is essentially the affirmation of existence.
— Nietzsche

Many of us who have been slaves to our addiction don't seem to have much energy left to affirm the joy of being alive. Our fantasies and acting out were so absorbing that we became almost like sleepwalkers. The images that obsessed us left little room for reality, as we daydreamed our way through life.

As we recover, we need to find new directions for our energy and new orientations for our affections. We will find ourselves wanting to reach out and affirm our hold on life.

Art can move and inspire us as we become creative in building lives that are full of energy and affirmation. New images and feelings will come flooding in to fill the spaces left by our old addictive fantasies. By participating in this flow of vitality we will find ourselves joining those artists and all others who say yes to life.

I am learning to use my newfound energy to be a creative force in the world and affirm the value of all life.

PW

. . . parts of you are still in unfinished business.
— *Julius*

And what do we do on the days when we feel nothing, when our hearts and minds are frozen and impenetrable? What kind of patience does it take to go through such a time without losing hope or faith? How do we endure until our feelings return?

Very gently. Emotions cannot be commanded to appear. When we do not feel, there is always a good reason. We can uncover it if we wish, but we must also be willing to wait. Sometimes there is nothing else to be done. If we can resist the urge to panic or over-rationalize, it's easier to be gentle with ourselves. If we can be flexible, being with people and being alone, depending on our needs, we will find balance. Above all, if we can stay abstinent, we will be peaceful. Feelings return when the time is right and we are ready to face, bear, accept, and welcome them.

My feelings are like a river flowing within me. I experience them, and I let go.

SK

Man is what he believes.

— *Anton Chekhov*

Practicing sex addicts act out of a perverted set of beliefs. This system convinces us we are worthless and shameful, and therefore our actions don't matter. In this way we were able to avoid taking responsibility for what we did, and we were not "there" within our own sexuality.

Sooner or later we found that our fantasies and acts didn't satisfy us. They were empty, ritual gestures that had no real human connection. We treated others as objects to gratify our own addictive desires so that nothing had any meaning beyond our self-serving fantasies.

In order to change our actions, we must change our beliefs. This is difficult to accomplish alone; we need to bounce our ideas off others. In a group where we are accepted and feel at home, we can try out new beliefs and develop new ways of relating to ourselves and to the world. We learn to change our values and our behavior, so that our addiction can be shed like an old skin.

I am beginning to change my beliefs so that my feelings can change about myself and my relationship with others.

PW

*No, this is not me, this is somebody else that
    suffers.*
*I could never face that, and all that has
    happened:*
Let sackcloth and ashes enshroud it,
And see all the lamps are removed...
    Night.

— Anna Akhmatova

We are people with needs. We're not different in this. But as sex addicts it's more likely some of our important needs were not met when we were children. Now we're adults, and the feeling of neediness is a chasm within us. And to make things harder, the child within us still feels ashamed because he or she needs.

Unless we help ourselves, our pain and shame will turn into rage, which only gives us the illusion of control. But rage empties us, and we cannot run on empty forever, trying to hide our true feelings.

Our needs are real, and we have nothing of which to be ashamed. Whether through reaching out to others in the program, turning to our Higher Power, or trusting our inner resources in quiet solitude, we can meet our own needs.

May I be gentle with my neediness. I do not have to be perfect, only real.

SK

*The principal mark of genius is not perfection
but originality, the opening of new frontiers.*
— *Arthur Koestler*

Many of us have been brought up to believe that we
should strive for perfection, and often this means im-
itating someone whose life seems exemplary to us. We
take enormously high standards from outside and we
soon begin applying them to ourselves.

When we fall short, we berate ourselves. We become
convinced that because we can't be saints, we must have
fallen from grace; imperfect, we come to despise ourselves. Surely, no one is as worthless as we are! We've
failed again, acted out. Who could possibly love us if
they knew who we really were?

But why do we insist on being judged by impossible
standards? Why do we want to be like someone else?
Why should we not search for what makes us original,
precious, and worthy of care and love? Then we don't
have to go around with our eyes on the ground; we can
look the world in the face because we know who we
are. Who? Ourselves.

---

*I don't want to be perfect. I want to be human. I want to
be myself.*

PW

One can never consent to creep when one feels an impulse to soar.

— *Helen Keller*

The risks we took as practicing addicts were profound. We took the chance that our spouse or others we cared about wouldn't discover the truth about our acting out. We juggled multiple relationships. We gambled we wouldn't get pregnant or pick up a sexually-transmitted disease. Our lives were built like a house of cards. We may not have called ourselves compulsive gamblers, but we were. We risked our very lives for the thrill of living dangerously.

In recovery we can channel our willingness to risk into constructive change. We can trust that what we do will help us grow; we can act and then let go of the outcome. Although it was our willingness to risk that got us into trouble, it is the same willingness that got us into recovery and keeps us there a day at a time.

Is my desire to do something that's risky coming out of my addiction or my recovery? An honest answer to that question will help me decide what to do.

SK

There is no humiliation for humility.
— *Joseph Roux*

When we were young we may have gone to someone for help and been met with coldness. Perhaps our friends mocked us when we tried to open up to them. Or, we were taken advantage of because we were sensitive and vulnerable. In short, we may have felt humiliated whenever we wanted to open up.

So we resolved not to let ourselves be open and dependent. We closed ourselves off from others and became grandiose in our belief that we could go it alone.

Now, in our recovery, we are learning to be humble. We have come to realize that nobody is an island, cut off from the world. We don't know all the answers. We need the help of those who really do want to reach out to us.

It's hard to be humble when we were so often humiliated, but we have to risk again reaching out to others; the rewards can be amazing. And it's great not to be alone.

I know I don't have to keep on feeling humiliated. Being humble is a sign of strength, not of weakness. Now, I experience new power in my relationships with others.

PW

In an honest man there is always something of a child.

— Martial

Why is it that sometimes we can talk about a problem and still not feel better? Usually, that's a sign to keep talking. As we go through a discovery process about something that's bothering us, it's possible that we have left out important information. Or we might not know how we feel — the words are there, but only on a rational, intellectual level. The hurt, sadness, anger, joy, or resentment are missing. Maybe we haven't been able to admit our feelings even to ourselves. That can be the hardest part of working through a problem, even harder than being honest with another person.

To be comfortable enough with our feelings to always know how we feel is a lifelong process, and one we will never perfect. But we know that the more honest we are with ourselves, the more accepting we'll be as well. That's a gift we can give ourselves every day.

Today I will allow my feelings to guide me to be more honest. I no longer have to keep secrets from myself or others.

SK

The problem of the individual is not clarified by stressing the antagonism between the individual and society, but by stressing their mutual reinforcement.

— Ruth Benedict

Since the time of Romanticism, with its emphasis on the opposition between the artist and society, we have tended to stress the values of the individual over and against those of the social order. We speak much of individual will and freedom and less about ideas and ideals of community.

Perhaps that is why many of us feel so alone. Some of us, particularly if we're male, have been brought up to be independent, self-reliant, and competitive, and we may now find this a burden rather than a blessing.

We now have the chance to forge new bonds and create new relationships. Our Twelve Step program has carefully and deliberately evolved as a self-supporting community whose basis is mutual help and whose ethic is love, not competition. As we learn to live the program each day, we carry this message to others who may suffer from lives of isolation and destructive addiction.

I am proud to be a member of a group that prizes love and community above all else.

PW

There must be the listening ear, as well as the still small voice.

— God Calling

In the past when we needed help, our addiction to sex was the way we coped. It helped us escape, avoid reality, and manipulate people. Now that it's no longer an option, how do we begin to act differently?

Well, practice makes perfect; we can practice asking for help. We can start simply by staying aware of where we are vulnerable. Prying shame from its grip on our self-esteem helps. We can know that we do not have to live by different rules than other people; we don't have to be separate and isolated. We don't have to be perfect, only real. Asking for help is okay.

We have a Higher Power who will provide all the help we need, and provide answers that are beyond any human being to give. When we feel unable to reach out to others, even though we want to, we can take a risk and turn to our Higher Power. Turning to sex addiction never solved anything; turning to our Higher Power will.

I do not have to sacrifice my sanity in order to solve my problems; I can Let Go and Let God.

SK

We won't have a society if we destroy the environment.

— *Margaret Mead*

Our environment is everything that surrounds us and to which we are related. We do not exist separate from our environment but are part of it — a mutually supportive living universe.

We need to sense this relationship and to experience ourselves deeply as part of a healthy world. Our sex addiction prevents us from this, because it isolates us from the world and leads us into self-absorption and misery where we just don't care.

Recovery means building new relationships, making new connections, getting in touch with ourselves and with the beauty of everything that surrounds us. Let's move outward and explore and cherish the world in which we live. We belong there and need to nurture it as well as ourselves. Recovery gives us the energy to reach out and care.

Let's work together for healthy relationships in a healthy environment where we feel at home.

PW

October

We're talking roots and wings; love that is
magnetic enough to hold, yet magnanimous
enough to allow for flight.
— *Charles R. Swindoll*

This is for the day when you realize you can't stand your spouse or partner one more minute. It's for the time when everything inside urges a prompt, preferably permanent, retreat.

The statement, "No one ever said a relationship is easy" is an understatement for a sex addict. We must slow down and take care of ourselves during a difficult time with someone we love. We can take inventory of our thoughts and feelings. We can make a contract not to do something impulsive. We can step back and view our problems with humor.

Somewhere inside you is love and a commitment to your partner. This love and commitment are real, no matter how exasperating, bewildering, or undeserving he or she seems to be right now. Say to yourself, "This, too, shall pass," because it will.

I will ask for balance, humility, patience, and detachment
when I am having relationship problems.

SK

There must always be a struggle between parent and child, while one aims at power and the other at independence.
— *Samuel Johnson*

How sad it is when we cannot separate from our parents or they from us. Many of us failed to experience the process of separation as adolescents because our families, addicted and dysfunctional, couldn't let us go. Or we had already turned to sex addiction, and this sapped our time and energy. We were diverted from maturing when we should have been free to explore the ideas that help us mature.

So here we are, grown-up, maybe still trying to leave parents who should have turned our old bedroom into a home office long ago. What we have to offer our parents as adults is different from what we offered them as children. Not better, just different. Now, in recovery, we long to share the attributes of maturity we have struggled to achieve: wisdom, judgment, emotional balance, compassion, skills. But we cannot change our parents; we can only detach with love and ask God to care for them and bring them into recovery if that's what is best for them.

Everything within me is worth cherishing, both the childlikeness and the adult maturity.

SK

*Most of the evils of life arise from man's being
unable to sit still in a room.*

— *Pascal*

Many of us have been alone too long, and it is good
and healthy that we now reach out and join new communities. We need human interaction to break the spell
of our fantasies which can too easily take over our lives.
Our spirituality develops by reaching out and making
contact with others.

At the same time, we need to spend time alone. It is
often in solitude that we gain contact with ourselves and
with our Higher Power. We see ourselves as part of
something greater than ourselves, and that is healthy
and necessary for our recovery.

We need to develop the patience to bear with ourselves in solitude without resorting to fantasy and acting out. We need our own space and time alone. Solitude
is different from isolation or loneliness. It is often in
solitude that we are most creative, and sane.

*I am learning to welcome the quietness and fullness of
solitude.*

PW

No one else can set your boundaries for you.
— *Lois J.*

One way to create boundaries with people is to establish priorities in our relationships. In the past, out of loneliness and neediness, we may have talked to anyone, whether the person wanted to listen or not. In the mixed-up world of sex addiction, we often withheld our true feelings from people close to us, but perhaps spilled them to the clerk at the bank.

As we grow in self-esteem, our relationships improve and we act to meet our needs. Then we have a better sense of who we are. We make choices in our relationships and take responsibility for them. We learn to bear the pain of boundaries that aren't respected and enjoy the serenity of those that are.

We no longer need to give ourselves away in bits and pieces; we know now what it is to feel whole. We can simultaneously have acquaintances, friends, co-workers, and intimate relationships, both sexual and nonsexual, in our lives. We can trust we will act appropriately and that our boundaries will keep us safe.

Boundaries are set one person at a time. Today, I will celebrate my ability to know where I stand in relation to others.

SK

It is better to light a candle than to curse the darkness

— *Chinese proverb*

Usually, when we are down, we think only of our own lives and get angry at ourselves or at our fate. We feel cut off from the world and lost in a dark night that seems to have no end.

If we stay alone when we are hurt and sad, we will probably continue to be lost in darkness. We can spin our thoughts round and round ourselves until we lose contact with the lives of others, and our darkness deepens.

But when we take a step out of ourselves and become part of a loving, caring, supportive group, we find at once that we are not alone. We're reminded that others suffer too — from addiction, loneliness, shame, sickness, abandonment, bereavement. As they share their feelings with us and we with them, together we find the courage and strength to get through the darkness. And together we discover the dawn of a new day.

I know I can find strength and love by lighting a candle of hope with others in my Twelve Step group.

FW

*What the explorers before me have learned is
this: Human strength lies not in resistance, but
in giving. The key to prayer is simple surrender
and acceptance.*

— Will Steger

It's necessary to block out the noise of the world and
our own thoughts in order to be able to listen. And to
what do we want to listen?

There's a voice within us, different for each of us, that
calls us. But just as it's hard to have a conversation with
someone who does all the talking, so it's hard for our
Higher Power to respond to us if we never listen. Luckily,
God gives us ways to hear. We have our hearts, our
minds, our wills, our imaginations, our emotions, our
memories. All these open us to prayer.

It can be expedient to think of prayer as mere words
we say without caring what happens next. But the
spiritual life challenges us to more. To pray simply and
to listen humbly opens us to God's response. And, in
the end, isn't that what the human heart longs for?

I will speak to You today, God, and listen for Your response.

SK

Kindness it is that brings forth kindness always.
— *Sophocles*

Why are people sharp with me? Why does everyone look gloomy today? What's wrong with the world?

Why do we blame the world when we are out of sorts? Life, after all, is neutral. It is our moods and attitudes that affect our view of things and the responses we receive. If we are seeing life through the dark glasses of melancholy, then we can't blame the world for seeming grim.

When we are at ease with ourselves and feel at home in our lives, other people will seem friendly and serene. A smile will prompt a smile; a greeting will bring a friendly response. And when I am considerate with my neighbor, it sets good deeds in motion. Kindness, like laughter, is contagious.

I really do believe that it is kindness and love that make the world a brighter, better place.

PW

*The world was always yours; you would not
take it.*
— Archibald MacLeish

It's possible during a difficult time to become side-
tracked in self-pity, anxiety, anger, or fear. It can be
easier to do that than to look honestly at our responsibilities today. When we feel ourselves spiraling down,
possibly into our addiction to sex, it's time to ask some
hard questions.

What will I choose today? Am I willing to take care
of myself before I take care of anyone or anything else?
Is there a Step I can work, something I can do to stay
connected to my recovery program?

The answers are within us. We have infinite inner
resources and potential. We have people to whom
we can reach out. We have our Higher Power, and
we have a commitment to ourselves. Through all of
these, we will find the hope and encouragement we
need, just for today.

---

*I may feel like I'm swimming against the tide, and that's
all right. All I have to do is my best.*

SK

Dreams are the touchstones of our characters.
— Henry David Thoreau

Touchstones were used to test metal, marking the difference between what was base and what was precious. If we are attentive to our dreams, we may find they help us separate the meaningful from the worthless so that we can better understand our values.

Dreams often carry overt or hidden messages about our lives and our hopes and fears. As we recover, we become attentive to these messages that can become the touchstones of our recovery. Dreams can help us distinguish between what we really want and what our addiction has convinced us that we can't do without.

At times, our dreams may be fearful and distressing. We may find ourselves back in our addiction or in the unhappiness of our childhood. But we don't have to be afraid; sex addiction is part of our history, and yet it needn't play an active, destructive role in our present lives...unless we let it. We are free, after all, to move forward and change our lives. And as we do, we find our dreams are changing too.

I welcome my dreams and I see in them texts that teach me about my life.

PW

To live and let live, without clamor for distinction or recognition; to wait on divine Love; to write truth first on the tablet of one's own heart — this is the sanity and perfection of living, and my human ideal.

— Mary Baker Eddy

So much of recovery is simply routine. We make a choice, and then we make it again. Unlike the uncontrolled life of a practicing sex addict, life now has the sanity that comes from making good choices until they become new habits. Everything in us may rebel at this. Our addiction will tell us that a sane life is boring and mundane. But it's not: it frees us because it's manageable.

It's the small choices that count. Maybe we change the movies we see or the music we listen to. Maybe we eat lunch at work, rather than use a stolen lunch hour to act out. Maybe we take in an extra meeting before going on a date.

All we have to do is choose for these twenty-four hours, One Day at a Time. We can use the Serenity Prayer to help us. The bottom line is willingness, humility, and tenacious faith.

I will try to see day-to-day routines as giving me the sanity and stability I need to feel safe.

SK

*Speech is civilization itself.... It is silence
which isolates.*

— *Thomas Mann*

Often, when we're tempted to act out, we find that
speaking to another human being breaks the spell of
our obsession and returns us to the real world. Our
addiction thrives on secrecy and a trance-like silence,
and on the lack of communication and constructive
criticism from other people.

In our groups we learn to find words that express our
hurts, our solitude, our anxiety, and our degradation.
We may go back deep into our past and talk things over,
so that they become seen and heard by ourselves and
others. Language brings things out into the open. Words
can be revealing, persuasive, and healing.

We need to talk — to talk about things, to talk things
over, to talk things out. Through speech we relate to
others and become part of the human community.

*I am finding words to put me in touch with myself and make
contact with others.*

PW

Time cools, time clarifies; no mood can be maintained quite unaltered through the course of hours.

— *Thomas Mann*

It's good to occasionally ask ourselves, "How do I feel right now, this moment? Am I confused, angry, discouraged? Am I hopeful, happy, content? Am I all of these or more?" No matter what our emotional state is, we belong there. The present is always the right place to be.

When we came into recovery, our emotional vocabulary may have been limited by our addiction to sex. But now we see how wonderful it is to have a range of emotions. We can be indignant, frustrated, irritated, perplexed, joyful, curious. We can be vulnerable, defensive, cautious, trusting, strong, confident, or ambivalent. And that's just the beginning.

We get all the time we need; it takes time to become familiar with our emotional terrain. When we're aware of how we feel, we can accept ourselves as we are and we can give ourselves to the moment.

Part of my prayer and meditation today can be an honest look at my emotional state. Step Ten will help me.

SK

It is we that are blind, not Fortune.
— *Sir Thomas Browne*

Denial is one of the hardest parts of our illness to overcome. It is because many of us deny our addiction, and our addiction thrives on denial.

We deny we are ill if we project our behavior onto someone else or something outside ourselves. We may have said, "My mother stifled me and that's why I sometimes act out with prostitutes." Or, "I can't help my compulsive behavior; it runs in the family." Or, "It's fate, it's my destiny to be different." If we say things like this, we not only deny our conduct, we deny our responsibility. And that prevents us from seeking help and getting well.

Denial is like a web that entangles us and keeps us from being free and from making choices. We need to accept responsibility without feeling shame; we need to make a "fearless moral inventory of ourselves," and then articulate the good and bad points of our character. Only if we remain blind to ourselves will we remain in bondage to our addiction.

I want to get to know myself and accept responsibility for the good and bad things in my life.

PW

In me there is darkness But with you there is light.

— *Dietrich Bonhoeffer*

A speaker at a meeting said, "To continue something when I'm making mistakes takes emotional courage." She was talking about making a decision to turn her will and life over to her Higher Power, and how it works in her life. To keep turning our wills and our lives over to God's care moves us into unknown territory. We will make mistakes, which is why we need God's care as we experience it in the Third Step.

It's hard to keep going after we stumble, especially when we keep stumbling over and over again. With sexual abstinence comes the clarity and awareness to look honestly at ourselves and our mistakes. We want to stop making them. We want to be perfect. We're impatient to change. But change doesn't work that way. Instead, a caring God cushions us when we fall, loves us without conditions, and gives us everything we need. If God can forgive us when we make a mistake, how can we not do the same?

If I fall today, I will fall into the arms of my Higher Power. And then I'll get up again.

SK

*Do not make yourself so big, you are not
so small.*

— *Jewish proverb*

Many of us are so used to being competitive that, even
when there is nothing at stake, we exaggerate our qualities and boast of our accomplishments. We sometimes
display what we may call a "grandiose ego" — preten-
tious and false. This is particularly true of sex addicts
because we often feel the need to hide behind an in-
flated image of ourselves. Why? Because we're afraid of
being found out. We think we can prevent people from
knowing all about us.

As we move into recovery we find that we gain insight and confidence about ourselves. We are no longer
shame-based people, and so we don't need to hide behind a mask. Our sexuality is now ours to delight in
and not a source of fear and shame. We gain a sense
of proportion in our lives and a viable perspective on
who we are.

We are now neither angels nor beasts, and we can
be proud to be human.

*I am glad to be at a place where I can be fully human,
whether I'm alone or with others.*

PW

*Thou are not idle; in thy higher sphere, thy
spirit bends itself to loving tasks.*
— *James Russell Lowell*

Since many of us are children of sex addicts, alcoholics,
or parents with other addictive or abusive behaviors,
we may have learned early in life how to hold back,
how to move with caution, how to hedge our bets. We
learned, as well, to react instead of act. The bold, well-
thought-out action was not for us. We were impulsive.

As recovering adults we still learn by watching others,
but we don't need to act like the cautious, yet impulsive
child. We can choose to act as adults, deciding when to
act and when to wait. There is much to be learned and
there are new role models to help us. Our sponsor,
healthy friends, and our brothers and sisters in the program are on our side. We can ask questions, bring our
fears and concerns out into the open, and trust our ever-
growing wisdom. We can be vulnerable and still feel safe.

---

*Today, I will acknowledge my fear if I feel it, reassure the
child within me, and Let Go and Let God.*

SK

There is only one meaning of life, the act of living itself.

— *Erich Fromm*

Perhaps we spend too much time looking for the meaning of life, as if it were a formula that would grant us wisdom and power and happiness. Maybe there isn't a simple meaning to life, or just one meaning for everyone.

In our addiction, we felt there must be an answer, a single answer to all our problems. A magic formula, perhaps, that would cure us instantly and set us free. How we wanted someone to come and give us that formula!

But if there were a single answer, then life would be the same for everyone. And how boring that would be. What we learn in recovery is that life takes on meaning for each one of us only through our own actions and process of living — and that's what makes our lives unique and adventurous.

I'm glad to be engaged in a lifetime search for meaning.

PW

For, although it is true that fear and despair can overwhelm us, hope cannot be purchased with the refusal to feel.

— *Susan Griffin*

Most of us have slips in our recovery. It's true that the stronger our abstinence is, the further we get from the possibility of slipping. But being human as well as powerless over our sex addiction make slips a reality we all have to face.

We can be honest if we slip, both with ourselves and with others in the program. They, along with our Higher Power, will understand how we feel. We need never bear alone the remorse, alienation, and shame we feel after acting out. We can also resist the impulse to anesthetize ourselves with alcohol or something else to avoid the pain of a slip. Through the program we've learned how to make amends, especially to ourselves. We can put this knowledge to work again if we slip.

While a slip is painful, it's not a reason to fall back to where we started. Instead, we can recommit ourselves to sanity and manageability, letting go of the past and being abstinent today.

My abstinence exists from this moment on. I can handle the present and find sanity here and now.

SK

*Doubt is not a pleasant state but certainty is
a ridiculous one.*

— Voltaire

In recovery it is easy to become too sure of ourselves.
We talk things over in the group, fix our boundaries,
have a period of abstinence, and then think we can just
experiment a little. . .just once. . .to prove we are still
"in control."

Pride comes before a fall, indeed. And pride is often
simply the certainty that we are always right. We become
grandiose in our excessive sureness, and then have slips
that frighten us and threaten our recovery.

There is nothing wrong with a healthy dose of doubt.
There are lots of things we're not sure of, and we can
admit them honestly. Doubt can be a way of arriving
at the truth, and it certainly is a good antidote to
overconfidence.

---

*I see the danger of pride and I am taking the steps to move
ahead in my recovery.*

PW

Then through the thunderous silence, we may be able to hear a still, small voice, and words will be born anew.

— *Madeleine L'engle*

A recovering sex addict described his isolation like this: "I used to walk into my apartment at the end of the day and be acutely aware that no one was there. I wanted to cry because I felt so lonely. It never occurred to me that I wasn't alone — because I was there."

There's a difference between being alone and being isolated. Learning how to be alone is a risk, but it's worth taking. When we are content with what we're doing, solitude restores us. Looking out the window at a tree is productive if it nurtures us.

We find out who we are by spending time alone. It gives us the chance to think, to dream, to talk with our Higher Power. It enables us to know the wonder of who we are. Alone, we can experience self-acceptance, direction, wisdom, and peace. Alone, we can be created anew. But to isolate is to risk self-destruction. Which will it be today?

I will take time for myself today. I need not fear to be alone because I never am.

SK

The only true hope for civilization — the conviction of the individual that his inner life can affect outward events.

— Stephen Spender

Our addiction may have left us little time to think about our society and our world. We may have spent vast sums of money and energy feeding the disease that was devouring us. And the world was reduced to the fantasies that were spinning around in our heads.

We deserve better for ourselves. And we can change. There is a relationship between what we think and what we do — and what we do affects others as well as ourselves. Our addiction has caused misery to others. Our recovery brings joy to other people as well as to ourselves.

Changing our inner lives, becoming free from the stranglehold of addiction, releases new energy and desires which, turned outwards, act upon the world. We take and take again these Twelve Steps and spread the news of hope and recovery to others. We join in activities in the group and find ourselves growing spiritually. As we follow the path, we realize that we can and do make a difference by helping others live out their full potential.

I am not an island but part of a community that is affected by my beliefs and actions.

PW

As long as there is still so much noise inside,
so long will it be hard for others to approach
you, except for those who look deeper and feel
the undertow, the life-current that never stops.
— Etty Hillesum

There's a difference between forcing ourselves to act
and self-discipline. Self-discipline comes from within.
With it we feel the push to do something worthwhile, no
matter how small. Forcing ourselves to do something, on
the other hand, usually reflects an authority outside ourselves. We might make a point of getting to work on
time because our boss says we have to, not because we
want to. Or, we might go to meetings because our sponsor says that's good, not because it's what we've chosen.

Forcing ourselves may produce results, but for a sex
addict, it's not healthy. It reinforces our desire to rebel
and have our own way. Letting go of our belief in willpower lessens the need to set up forces outside ourselves to resist. Somewhere inside of us, even if it's faint,
is the sense of what's best for us, of what we truly want
to do. We may fight it, but our heart knows. And that's
the right choice. To follow what's in our heart teaches
self-discipline and brings self-esteem.

Joy, pleasure, and serenity are mine each day when I stay
centered and self-disciplined.

SK

To love without criticism is to be betrayed.
— *Djuna Barnes*

We talk about unconditional love, and we may think it means love without hassle. But where there is real love there is going to be conflict, because that is part of being truly human.

When someone we love criticizes us, we may be afraid. We may think we are going to lose that person because we are unworthy; we may turn against ourselves and then against our love.

But as we come to believe in ourselves and discover humility through our recovery, we can acknowledge our need for advice and helpful criticism. We don't have to be afraid of another's opinion. Criticism, lovingly offered, can help us see things in a new way. Love doesn't have to be blind; it can be clear-sighted, honest, and sincere.

I am learning to accept myself as I am, and I can take criticism from those who know me and love me.

PW

The possibilities for tomorrow are usually beyond our expectations.

— *Anonymous*

When it is struggle to believe that we're hopeful, productive, and capable of caring for and loving others, we may have to pretend that we are all of these things. The program calls this *acting as if.* We can act as if we're hopeful; we can act as if we're productive; we can act as if we care. We may not have a long record of being all these things, and we may not even know how sometimes, but we don't have to. We have a promise that our Higher Power is caring for us and will help us do the things we can't do on our own.

Acting as if is hard work; it takes constant letting go. We may feel totally unqualified to live in reality and resentful that we have to. Our grandiosity whispers that reality is boring and beneath us. We are "special"; we don't have to follow the same rules other people do.

Consciously turning our wills and our lives over to God stills the addictive voice and focuses our energy on real life. We become part of life, rather than an adversary. And we feel the pleasure of our efforts.

If today is a day to act as if, I will accept it and do my best.

SK

Grief can take care of itself, but to get the full value of joy, you must have someone to divide it with.

— Mark Twain

As sex addicts, many of us lost our ability to share joy with others. We may still rarely feel joy by ourselves and are frightened to let go with other men and women. We may have thought we were behaving freely when we were acting out, but we've realized that we were driven by our compulsion and bound by our obsessions. Expressing emotion spontaneously and freely is difficult.

In our group we learn to be honest about ourselves and open with others. "Thanks for sharing!" How many times do we hear those words as we learn to interact with others in the group? Soon we are laughing and crying — finding pleasure and release in letting go.

And now when we see footprints in the sand, a duck splash down onto the water, a jet take off, a windsurfer glide by, a child pucker up and snort with laughter, we can turn to our friends and share in the delight of the moment. We come to see how rich life can be when we share its simple pleasures with those we love.

It feels good to let go and share my delight with someone I love.

PW

Everything in Nature contains all the powers
of Nature. Everything is made of one hidden
stuff.

— *Ralph Waldo Emerson*

Power — what it is and how to use it — often raises
fears and questions for sex addicts. We all need to feel
power in our lives. But if, through abuse or never having been taught about power, we were deprived of our
personal power as children, we cannot magically possess it as adults.

As practicing sex addicts, we craved power and used
our addiction to get it. Our addiction was a plea for the
mastery of ourselves and our lives, something that all
humans need. We simply didn't know how to accomplish that honestly. But we can learn, starting today. We
can reject the kind of power that doesn't work and seek
the kind that does.

True power is creative, rather than destructive. It's
loose and flexible, not rigid. It does not need the ego.
It is a spiritual quality we possess, rather than an
authority over others that somebody endows us with.
When we look inside, our power is there, waiting for
us to find it.

The First Step helped me learn what powerlessness is. The
other Steps will help me create power that produces growth.

SK

What is most beautiful in virile men is something feminine; what is most beautiful in feminine women is something masculine.
— Susan Sontag

Some of us may be afraid of the other sex in us. Men, especially, often despise the feminine in themselves and do everything they can to put on a "macho" air. Women, too, are not always comfortable with what is masculine in themselves.

Many poets, philosophers, and psychologists believe that each of us is a complex mixture of the masculine and the feminine. We suppress either at our peril. What we dislike or close ourselves off to in the opposite sex may be just the qualities in ourselves that we fear the most.

Part of becoming whole means accepting the generous heritage of both sexes. In our recovery, we can get in touch with the feminine and the masculine in ourselves and other people. We will find our lives more complete if we do.

I embrace the whole of myself with affection and wonder.

PW

This pain is never permanent.
> — *Teresa of Avila*

Many of us have felt the impulse to pick up the phone and make the wrong call. You know the one. It's not that we want to; we don't. We can tell ourselves, as one group member did, "This could be dialing pain." But no matter what we do, eventually we will face the moment when it's just us and the phone. And it draws us like a magnet.

We must be willing to go to any lengths at such a time. To make that first phone call can lead anywhere, especially to a slip. The program gives us the tools we need, especially the first three Steps. We can call someone from our group instead of someone who is part of our sex addiction. We can choose abstinence one minute at a time, if necessary. We may feel alone with our fear, loneliness, and compulsion, but we're not. With our Higher Power's help, we will emerge safely, with our abstinence undamaged.

God, help me meet moments of compulsion with patience, willingness, and courage.

SK

*The usual drawback of success is that it annoys
one's friends so.*

— P. G. Wodehouse

Some of us really do fear success, partly because of
the responsibility. But often the real reason is that we
still do not feel worthy.

As practicing sex addicts we feared disclosure. We
often shunned the spotlight and led obscure, desperate
lives. We may still tend to flee success because we might
be subject to scrutiny. . .and perhaps be unmasked.
Others would see us as we really are — or as we are
afraid we are. And we are so used to thinking of ourselves as failures that we don't see how we could possibly earn or deserve success. So how can we win?

We need to remind ourselves that we don't have to
fall back into our old, self-defeating attitudes. In recovery
we can't sustain these attitudes; our new friends won't
let us. Gradually, we find we are moving away from fear
of failure and fear of success. As our self-esteem grows,
we become more confident in our abilities to live a
productive and joyful life.

*I am beginning to feel happy and successful in whatever
I choose to undertake.*

PW

What we love we shall grow to resemble.
— Bernard of Clairvaux

There comes a day when we realize that looking for external solutions to our problems will not work. How vain has been the time and energy spent looking for the perfect mate, the perfect job, the perfect life. So, instead, we start to search for internal solutions. We begin to change ourselves.

To change ourselves is a different process from controlling ourselves, which cannot be done. But when we start to give up the control, the rigidity, the perfectionism, the self-will, we begin to change. This change seems like a miracle because it is. It's an incredible gift from our Higher Power, who loves us beyond our imagining. The more we change our focus from the external to the internal, the more we're able to accept ourselves. We become humble with each small choice to accept ourselves as we are. We become whole as we let that choice be enough for today.

Am I living within myself or outside myself today? To keep the focus within requires self-acceptance.

SK

To be able to fill leisure intelligently is the last product of civilization.

— *Arnold Toynbee*

Some of us have a lot of time to devote to things other than work. If we allow our addiction to fill up this time — as it so easily can — then we become tired and wretched. There is nothing more time-consuming or more exhausting than an obsession.

As we recover we find that we have more time at our disposal for leisure and play. We can take time to visit friends and loved ones, to go outdoors, to develop hobbies, to play sports, and to look at and listen to all the fine and exciting things that surround us.

Time off is necessary, and it becomes invigorating if we bring to it new energy and purpose. We are changing and we feel grateful to our Higher Power for a new sense of serenity and purpose. We can now play openly and joyfully in harmony with the wonders of living.

My time away from obsession is time to live and love as a free person.

PW

November

It is not yours to finish the task, but neither are you free to take no part in it.
— *Anonymous*

Nearly every time we make a choice, we let go of something else. When we feel unsure of what to do, we can ask ourselves whether one choice is more positive than the other: "Which will help me feel good about myself? What does my heart tell me to do?" We can allow ourselves not to expect perfection, but to do the best we can — and let go. Each honest choice increases our self-esteem, our faith in our ability to change, and our willingness to keep working.

Do you remember your first meeting? From that moment, perhaps, you were no longer alone; you had reached common ground by joining with a group of people who had each made a choice to recover. Getting into recovery may have been the most powerful statement of self-love you had ever made.

We found the program, we stay with it, and we work it every day. We are truly marvels of courage and fidelity, shining examples of God's infinite respect for our choices.

Whether small or large, my choices today matter. I will give each one my best.

SK

We can destroy ourselves by cynicism and dis-
illusion just as effectively as by bombs.
— Kenneth Clark

In some circles it is considered smart to be cynical
and hypercritical. There may have been times when we
tried to make ourselves look tall by diminishing everything around us, by not being "taken in." We acted as
if we had seen and done it all before, as if we were above
everything, the ones who were really with it.

In recovery, we have begun to wake up to the myriad
splendors of the world around us. We've discovered that
we aren't too jaded to admire a sunset, too sophisticated
to let ourselves go on the dance floor, too old and tired
to respond to a child's laughter. Our example affects
others, especially our children. We no longer want to
taint their vision of the world through our indifference
and our jeering.

May we keep our vision fresh and open to the wonder
of everyday life. We are in the world not to scoff and
sneer but to appreciate the beauty and diversity of life.

I'm learning to love being here, and want to affirm my belief
in the richness and goodness of the world.

PW

A word fitly spoken is like apples of gold in pictures of silver.

— Prov. 25:11

Facing our own dishonesty can be daunting, but maintaining absolute honesty is a basic premise of our recovery program. The Big Book describes it as "rigorous" honesty, and for sex addicts, it starts with abstinence. To believe we can be honest without a solid commitment to abstinence simply won't work.

The more we grow, the more we develop our ability to make one choice at a time, to experience one feeling at a time, to tell the truth one situation at a time. We admit to ourselves when we feel guilty, angry, fearful, resentful — the negative feelings that are difficult to face. Being honest is how we finally come to know what used to baffle us about our addiciton. When we create a unity between honest feeling, honest thinking, and honest action, we find that we have become honest people.

Personal honesty is a gift of my recovery for which I thank God every day.

SK

If any thing is sacred, the human body is sacred.

— *Walt Whitman*

Whitman, one of our great poets, sang the delights of the quick and vibrant body. We are not split into container and content but we are unified and whole. We need to feel ourselves in our bodies alive.

Sex addiction stunts and maims us. We become humiliated by our sexuality and ashamed of our bodies. We may become sick, even diseased. When we act out, we are not united but split into different parts. And we watch ourselves betray our humanness. Obsessive sexual behavior turns us into people only half alive.

We have begun to return to a full sense of ourselves. This we do as we speak openly and fearlessly of our addiction and enter into new relationships with our Higher Power, other people, and ourselves. We find that this new sense of ourselves includes good feelings about the integrity of our bodies, fully alive.

As I change, let me take note of my growing sense of the integrity of my body.

PW

"Here," she said, "in this place, we flesh; flesh that weeps, laughs; flesh that dances on bare feet in grass. Love it. Love it hard."
— Toni Morrison

Our body belongs to us, is a part of who we are. It is us, just as our intellect, spirit, and feelings are part of us. As sex addicts, we often have a love-hate relationship with our body. We often disconnect from our body — especially when we're being sexual — in order not to feel pain. To disconnect from any part of ourselves hurts. Like walking on a sprained ankle, we compensate as best we can, but part of us is missing; part of us isn't working the way it's supposed to. And that part is our sense of ourselves as physical beings.

Recovery means reclaiming our body. We start from where we are and form a new relationship with ourselves. We can do it by changing our eating habits, exercising, improving our personal grooming, and going to the doctor. We patiently fill in the missing pieces of nurturing and attention. Then our sense of ourselves as whole people will include our newfound love of our body.

I have only one body. It was given to me not to misuse, but to love and care for.

SK

*One of the signs of passing youth is the birth
of a sense of fellowship with other human
beings as we take our place among them.*
— *Virginia Woolf*

When we were young many of us were intent on
moving forward and cultivating our talents and skills,
sometimes in a competitive arena, but often alone. In
our society it is the development of the individual that
is stressed in childhood and adolescence. As a result,
many of us grow up feeling isolated.

Some of us remain alone. We don't manage to find our
place in a community, or we don't find the community
that suits us. And if we are addicts, we withdraw into
our own worlds of self-satisfaction and self-concern,
where we become armored against other people.

One of the challenges and rewards of working in a
Twelve Step program is the opportunity to live, work, and
grow with other people, sharing their hopes, fears, needs,
and desires. We begin to see that what really matters,
even beyond individual talent, is fellowship and love.

---

*I am grateful for the opportunity to stand outside myself
and join with others in the adventure of recovery.*

PW

The readiness is all.

— *William Shakespeare*

Willingness is like faith. We know it's real because we experience it, but we can't define it. Nonetheless, the sense of humility, surrender, and peace that accompany willingness are our indicators that it is real, indeed.

A recovering addict who had recently finished treatment told this story: "I was walking downtown and I got at least three offers to buy drugs or sex. I said no. My willingness at that moment was to say no."

We move forward often without knowing where we're going. But in those rare, shining moments of willingness when we conform our will to God's, we see our direction clearly. And we are transformed.

May my willingness, like my faith, become stronger as I surrender to my Higher Power.

SK

Let your tears come. Let them water your soul.
— *Eileen Mayhew*

We often want to sit down and cry, but the tears don't seem to come. For years we may have struggled to keep ourselves from crying, because we've been made to feel that tears are a sign of weakness. And we certainly don't want to look foolish and vulnerable in front of our "tough" friends!

One of the good things about joining and building trust with a group of other people recovering from sex addiction is that we can let down our defenses and not feel exploited. We can show our tenderness for others and ask to be cared for. Our addiction has kept us aloof from others, but now we can begin to get close. We know we are safe now and among people who know what it means to trust and love again.

So when the tears feel like coming, we can now let them come. What a relief it is to weep for the hurt child within us or cry over a painful separation. Tears help us mourn our losses and bring us in touch with the present.

I am no longer afraid to show my emotions. I share my experiences in tears and laughter.

PW

Happiness is not a state to arrive at, but a manner of traveling.
— Margaret Lee Runbeck

We all want to be happy. When we're not, we try to figure out why. We think about it, and perhaps go into therapy or add another meeting. We blame ourselves, blame our parents, blame our sex addiction — but we're still not happy.

Being happy is exactly that: a state of being. We all know the difference between acting happy and being happy; we spent years acting happy because we thought that's what people expected. When we were practicing sex addicts, looking at happiness from the other side of an unbridgeable chasm, we literally didn't know how it felt because we had rarely experienced it. But recovery gives us the example of happy people who teach us until, finally, we are able to teach ourselves.

I can be happy today. It may not be easy, and it probably won't be perfect, but even a moment's happiness is worth the effort.

SK

The important thing is not to stop questioning.
— Albert Einstein

We used to think we knew it all. We had grandiose ideas about ourselves. We stopped asking hard questions that could cause our fragile world of make-believe and deviousness to come crashing down. We protected our addiction by fleeing from the questions that could have started us on the road to recovery.

One day the questions flooded in unchecked. Why am I out of control? How come I can't look my beloved in the eye? Why don't I have time for my friends? Why do I get irritated with my children? Why do I feel so bad about myself, so filled with shame? Why can't I cope? Why is my life unmanageable?

Unmanageable? When we feel this question deeply, then we are already on the road to recovery, for we know we can't continue to go it alone. The question suggests an answer: we need others, a different system of support, a program of recovery, a Higher Power, serenity, love.

This is what we really wanted and needed, and this is what we find in our Twelve Step program.

Learning to be honest means continuing to ask questions about ourselves and our situation in the world.

PW

*Love alone is capable of uniting living beings
in such a way as to complete and fulfill them,
for it alone takes them and joins them by what
is deepest in themselves.*
— *Teilhard de Chardin*

Experiencing our sexuality once we've entered recovery presents many challenges. Once we've brought our addiction into the light, everything looks different, especially sex. One of the first things we learn is that we are always sexual beings, whether we're in a relationship or by ourselves.

Recovery doesn't mean renouncing our sexuality; indeed, it means embracing it in a new way. Our personal abstinence determines our behavior and helps us decide when it's appropriate to be sexual. We choose when or whether to be sexual with ourselves, and how to stay abstinent during a sexual experience. We have new values, support from others, the wisdom of the program, and our spirits to guide us. Through recovery we will learn to respect, nurture, and eventually love our sexuality just as we're learning to do for the other parts of ourselves.

I believe my sexuality is healing each day as I treat myself with gentleness.

SK

It is courage the world needs, not infalli-
bility. . .courage is always the surest wisdom.
— *Sir Wilfred Grenfell*

To overcome feelings of shame and to reorient our desires requires patience, support, and courage. We may be tempted to say to ourselves that the task is too difficult and that we are perfectly content to go on the way we are.

But wisdom tells us otherwise. Wisdom is that insight and knowledge we have gained for ourselves by beginning to live out our recovery. And wisdom tells us that we need to change and move out of our addiction. If we don't listen to this voice of wisdom, we waste our talents and our potential as human beings.

Wisdom is the insight and the perspective we gain on ourselves and the world. Courage is the action of changing our beliefs and behavior and helping others along the path. Together, wisdom and courage lead us to serenity and the knowledge that we are growing and living more fully and sanely day by day.

I need courage to change, and I will find it if I am wise enough to see the true benefits of recovery from addiction.

PW

In the darkest hour the soul is replenished and given strength to continue and endure.
— *Heart Warrior Chosa*

In the depths of our addiction to sex, some of us hated ourselves so much that we didn't believe we deserved to live. Some of us had this idea planted in our minds when we were children. Some of us had lives that didn't seem worth living. And some of us were suffering so much from our addiction that we were willing to do anything to be rid of it. When things are that hard, some of us turn to thoughts of suicide.

How do we go on when we can't any longer? Very gently. We use everything we can to help us stay alive: the thought of a beloved child, a friendship with a group member, time-out from our normal life, turning ourselves over to our Higher Power. When we feel suicidal, we may not care about anything; we feel alienated and isolated. But we're not. To even keep breathing connects us to life. And if we open ourselves to the fullness of the moment, from this most basic act our connections expand infinitely. We've only to hang on, one minute at a time, and reasons to hope again will come.

My life is precious because it was given to me by my Higher Power, who loves me.

SK

Passions are less mischievous than boredom, for passions tend to diminish and boredom increase.
— *Barbey d'Aurevilly*

One of the great modern diseases is boredom, and for many of us it is the ground of our sex addiction. When time is slow and heavy, we trip off into fantasies and obsessions. And the next step could be to act out. This mechanism can take so strong a hold on us that we may feel we can't do much to escape the vicious cycle of boredom and addiction.

But modern life is as rich, varied, and colorful as life was at any other time. Most of us who have our health are surrounded by all kinds of challenges and excitements. All we need to do is to move out into the world and use our senses. Thousands of delights await us.

Perhaps we need to take on a regular schedule of exercise, not necessarily anything strenuous or costly. A simple walk can work wonders. We'll learn to see the world as a real place and not merely through a film of fantasy. We gain energy by acting in the world; we lose it by acting out.

I need to plan my activities and move outward, into the world.

FW

To love human beings is still the only thing worth living for; without that love, you really do not live.

— *Sören Kierkegaard*

If we could save each other, we would be God. But we can't, and we're not God. We can, however, make a difference. We help set ourselves free from sex addiction by working for the freedom of others. Sometimes we must take a risk and break our anonymity in order to offer hope and understanding where there was none. Sometimes we must be silent and wait for God's time, even when everything within us is saying: Do Something. Sometimes there is nothing to be done. Often, suffering must be endured until a person decides not to suffer anymore, and only then does another path open up.

But that doesn't mean we can't offer our silent prayers for God's will to be done. That doesn't mean we can't be compassionate. We can listen even when we don't want to, offer the program even when it seems to fall on deaf ears, and best of all, offer the example of our own lives. When we detach, we join our will to God's and that's the best gift of all we can give.

If someone needs my help today, I will use Step Twelve to guide my actions.

SK

A man is known by the company his mind keeps.

— *Thomas Bailey Aldrich*

We are often judged by the friends we have, but perhaps we are also known by what we read and listen to and see at the movies and on television. Certainly, everything that happens to us affects us, and everything that affects us influences our way of dealing with other people and viewing the world.

Many sex addicts devour pornography, go to X-rated movies and watch "blue" videos. "It's harmless," we say. "We have a right in this country to see and hear what we like."

Freedom from censorship — that's an issue in itself. But as sex addicts we are particularly vulnerable to material that focuses narrowly on the human body as an object of lust and exploitation. As sex addicts, we tend, in any case, to dehumanize people and view sex as an act without consequences, divorced from intimacy. Exposure to material that insults sex increases our fixations, our isolation, our fantasies, and our shame.

There's so much to see and hear and savor in the world. Why demean ourselves with actions that only drive us deeper into shame and despair?

I need to open my mind to the wonders of life and knowledge.

*An act of love that fails is just as much a part
of the divine life as an act of love that succeeds,
for love is measured by its own fullness, not
by its reception.*

— Harold Loukes

It's the nature of love to create, and there is power
in each act of love, no matter how small. To choose to
forgive rather than to blame creates good and is, therefore, an act of love. To turn away from sex addiction and
stay abstinent accomplishes the same thing. And, unlike possessing something external that brings no
guarantee of happiness, creating good makes us happy.

For a sex addict, love is a word often accompanied
by pain and unfulfilled longing. When we've never
known love, it's a word and no more. We may have an
intellectual idea of love, but it remains an idea with no
reality if we've never experienced it.

Recovery allows us to more fully experience love, intimacy, tenderness, closeness, and warmth. At first, these
may be unfamiliar and difficult to allow or accept. But
if we remember that love creates only good, we will have
a sense of purpose and a reason to try.

*I am a good person. I am a loving person. Today, I will be
true to those beliefs about myself.*

SK

Praising what is lost
Makes the remembrance dear.
— *Shakespeare*

Many of us who are sex addicts view the past with regret or remorse; we miss it because of our pleasures or we feel guilty because of our trespasses. Our memories have us at center stage, which gives them a narrow, self-centered range.

As we meet with others and talk our way into a balanced view of ourselves, we are likely to revise our notions of the past. To our surprise and joy, we find our focus widening; we are taking in other people. We are no longer isolated figures, but part of a landscape thronged with family and friends.

One of the great things about our newfound health is this ability to recall an expanding past with pleasure and joy as we achieve a wider, more generous perspective. Our world grows and takes on more varied and deeper meanings.

Now I am sane again. I can expand my vision of the past and find much to love and praise there.

FW

What is moral is what you feel good after.
— Ernest Hemingway

For so long, we defined feeling good by short-lived, sensual gratification. One of the consequences of sex addiction is the weakening or, worse, near destruction of our moral values. Taking inventory of our morals in recovery helps us on our way to becoming truly moral people once again.

We can decide what our personal morals are through experience, the program's wisdom, and the guidance of a Higher Power. One of the greatest gifts of recovery is moral integrity, an inner and steadfast sense of what is right and wrong. If we do not have this, we will be forced to depend on things outside ourselves. If we espouse one thing publicly, but don't really believe it, we will not live it, either. Our recovery depends on consistent values — especially values about sexuality — that lets us feel serene and good about ourselves. With the help of a searching and fearless inventory, we can live now according to our personal sense of morality and truly feel good again.

I will be open to the ideas of other people, but I will be guided by my own values.

SK

If only God would give me some clear sign! Like making a large deposit in my name in a Swiss bank account.

— *Woody Allen*

It is not superstitious to believe that we will know what to do at times because of a voice within or a signal from without. A feeling, a dream, a presence, a word from a friend, a glance from a loved one — these can each be ways our Higher Power works in our lives.

Such signs may not be obvious, and they may not always seem immediately beneficial. When we accepted that our lives had become unmanageable, our first reaction may have been panic and hopelessness. What can we do? Why should the world care about me?

In reality the first two Steps of our program lead us to a new sense of spirituality. We admitted that we are powerless over our addiction and accepted a dependence on a Power greater than ourselves. And this is a major part of the road back to health.

Let's learn to read the signposts along the path to recovery. Let's take heart from the fact that we can be helped by forces outside ourselves, that we are not alone.

I realize that the world is full of signs that can help me understand myself and my path through life.

We only acknowledge small faults in order to make it appear that we are free from great ones.

— *La Rochefoucauld*

There is nothing quite so intimidating as taking a searching and fearless moral inventory of ourselves. It's no wonder we're tempted to avoid the challenge of this Step in our recovery. One way to make an inventory easier is to do it with the help of our Higher Power. To face ourselves as we are — and as we have been in the past — can be overwhelming unless we are sustained by God's unconditional love.

As we commit ourselves to self-knowledge, we will be grateful for what we learn in our inventory. Our fear will lessen. But even if we are afraid now, it's important to take the plunge and do the best we can. We do not have to wait until we are perfect, because that time will r:ever come. We can keep our inventory simple, doing it a bit at a time, or we can do it exhaustively, getting everything out. The point is to do it. We need not carry our character defects around like a sack of old, useless tools. We must be who we are today.

Taking inventory helps me heal the past, live in the present, and look forward to the future.

SK

One must not lose desires. They are mighty stimulants to creativeness, to love, and to long life.

— *Alexander Bogomoletz*

In sex addiction our desires became turned inward, toward our own gratification, without real regard for others. We closed ourselves off in worlds of fantasy where we alone were in control, and others became mere objects for our pleasure. We lost contact with the world.

Desires are healthy and potent forces for change, growth, and love. We can own our sexuality and not let it own us, so that we can reorient our desires toward loving action in the world.

For too long our desires have isolated us. We had become grandiose in our self-concern and in our refusal to let others into our lives. Recovery will bring a new focus for our sexual energy, and we will find not pain and weariness but joy and energy in our new relationships.

My desires are forces for change, love, and renewal.

FW

I will walk in God's presence, in the land of the living.

— Ps.116:9

Part of treating ourselves well is making sure we allow room for pleasure. Even though we may have misused our capacity for pleasure when we were acting out, we are not doomed to a life that's dull and sensationless now that we're abstinent. On the contrary, we can enjoy life even more as we expand our capacity for pleasure beyond the narrow bounds of our addiction.

There are all kinds of ways to bring healthy, respectful satisfaction into our lives. It might be physical activity, such as a good workout. It could be the pleasure of an hour spent in a creative activity. A conversation with a good friend is deeply satisfying.

We can move beyond the past when we may have associated pleasure principally with our addiction to sex. We realize now that all people need satisfaction and gratification. Being in recovery does not mean a life of total deprivation; it is a way of living that allows us to reach out to enjoy the things of real value life has to offer. When we're not ruled by fear, we can appreciate more of how truly pleasurable it is to be alive.

What pleasures will I find today that are mine for the asking?

SK

The novel is the perfect medium for revealing to us the changing rainbow of our living relationships.

— D. H. Lawrence

Our everyday life often becomes so predictable we become oblivious to variation in life. We establish connections with people and then perhaps take them for granted. Even in our intimate relationships we may not be aware of the changes taking place.

But change is the law of life. Nothing is static, least of all people. We see this when we read a well-written novel, where our vision of the characters is constantly shifting as they evolve and change during the story. From our privileged, objective position as readers we watch the ebb and flow of relationships as they develop and become different.

We can take this perspective into our own lives. We can become more attentive to the complexity and subtleties of our inner lives and our relationships with those we love. As we recover from our addiction, this can help us be open to the. new and the marvelous in our relationships.

I want to become attentive to change and renewal in everything around me, especially my relationships.

PW

Visions for those too tired to sleep.
These seeds cast a film over eyes which
*   weep.*

— Amy Lowell

Many of us have struggled with depression during our lives. Many of us have also felt shame when we were depressed, as if we were lazy or weren't trying hard enough.

But that isn't true. The causes of depression are complex, and those of us who suffer from it owe it to ourselves to keep searching for relief. As recovering addicts, we long to put all our energy into our new lives. The hopelessness, self-blame, and apathy of depression can be paralyzing and even life-threatening. In recovery, when we need to eliminate stress, depression is a burden we don't have to carry.

Whether our feelings are a result of external circumstances or our body's chemistry, we can take good care of ourselves. We can feel our anger and sadness. We can seek professional help if necessary. Recovery doesn't mean an end to suffering, but the program promises this too shall pass. There can be an end to the suffering of depression. We have good reason to hope we will feel joy again.

In my Higher Power's compassion for my suffering, I find strength and consolation.

SK

*I believe that a sign of maturity is accepting
deferred gratification.*

— *Peggy Cahn*

One of our problems as active sex addicts was our
inability to put off our own gratification. We lived in the
world of the Pleasure Ego where we imagined everything was at our beck and call. Closed off from reality
by our egoism, we thought we had to satisfy our desires
"right now," regardless of the consequences.

Reality includes other people, and they may not wish
to participate in our pleasure or respond to our demands.
They have their own lives to live and their own freedom of choice. For some of us, this brought on angry
tantrums where we lashed out verbally or even with
violence. We were so used to having our own way that
opposition quite literally maddened us.

We're learning in recovery that the world was not
created just for us. Its particularity and beauty is to be
enjoyed — but not just by us, not necessarily at this very
second. We now can wait, be patient, and respect the
desires of others, while enjoying the unfolding of our
Higher Power's design for us.

---

*I know I am still often selfish and impatient, but I am
learning to cherish mutuality in the world and respect other
people's freedom.*

PW

The price of dishonesty is self-destruction.
— *Rita Mae Brown*

We may believe that after having been dishonest about something small and seemingly inconsequential, we would be honest and make the right decision when faced with a more important issue. But real honesty comes from the hundred small choices we make every day.

It is easier to be honest when we are integrated: mind, body, spirit, and feelings working together. As sex addicts, we've all experienced the tug-of-war between our mind, feelings, body, and spirit. In our addictive behavior, we chose the part of us that called the loudest, usually our body.

Through the program we learn how to be honest and, gradually, we learn how to live as whole people. We can be free of shame, self-pity, self-righteousness, resentment — all the character defects that add up to dishonesty. Sex addiction affects the whole person and recovery does too. The first is inherently dishonest; the second offers integrity.

Each of the Steps shows me, in a different way, how to be honest. Which one do I need today to stay true to myself?

SK

What a wonderful life I've had! I only wish I'd realized it sooner.

— *Colette*

Colette was a French writer whose books give us a sense of a life fully lived. Yet, even she regretted that she hadn't appreciated her good fortune earlier on. It was only while writing that she learned to see how lucky and happy she was and to praise life.

Many of us are also tardy in realizing how rich our lives have been. It is often only in retrospect that we can see the beauty and feel the joy. How beautiful that day was! How much I was loved! How lucky I was to have such good friends around me! What a lovely child!

Why didn't we see what was happening in front of our very eyes? Why couldn't we seize the moment? It is good to remember, but it is also splendid to live in the present and cherish each moment while it is happening.

I am learning to let go and live in the intensity of the here and now.

PW

A decent boldness ever meets with friends.
— Homer

Serenity is the goal of our recovery, and to attain it we need both wisdom and courage. It is difficult to speak of courage out of context; but we know it when we feel it or see it. It often shows itself in little everyday acts just as much as in grand gestures.

We need courage in our daily struggle against our addiction. We need to be brave enough to face up to our disease. It will not go away just because we detest it; we need to take steps, every day — small, determined steps.

For this we need courage. And in our program we will see it every time we listen to a First Step or hear someone out in our small groups. We meet many brave people who admit their lives are unmanageable and who are taking steps to change.

Courage is contagious. When we see it, feel it, hear it, we are impressed, affected, energized. If we keep our eyes and ears open, we will see and hear about plenty of brave things happening in our groups. And our own actions, as we recover, will be among them.

I am glad I am in touch with brave people in my group; their courage inspires me to exercise my own.

PW

*Behavior which is superficially correct, but is
intrinsically corrupt always irritates those who
see beneath the surface.*
— *James Bryant Conant*

As sex addicts, our acting out was in many ways a
never-ending search for power. We sought power over
people so we could fulfill our compulsion for addictive
sex. We treated others as objects and felt powerful doing it. We looked at a world obsessed with sex, where
people misuse sex and power with impunity. And we
thought, if they can do it, so can I. That's addictive thinking, which leads only to illusory power.

We become truly powerful by learning to love ourselves and then acting that way. We become powerful
by turning ourselves over to our Higher Power.

Healthy power has been defined by Gershen Kaufman as making choices, living consciously, and being
responsible. Healthy power energizes us, helps us feel
good about ourselves, and centers us. We find this power
through simple choices that focus our attention inward,
on our honest needs. Then we practice using it, One
Day at a Time.

*Where is the source of my power today? I have a choice:
my addiction or my Higher Power.*

SK

December

Every beginning is a consequence — every beginning ends some thing.
— Paul Valéry

Recovery is a beginning, a rebirth, the dawn of a new life. It is not simply a miracle, which comes from heaven; it is the effect of our desire to change, to make our lives anew with the help of our Higher Power.

Our lives before recovery were unmanageable, and that knowledge was the start of our recovery. We knew we needed a new set of beliefs. Pursuing new beliefs is a part of our recovery.

Our recovery means the end of old ways of behaving. We may need to mourn the passing of our old selves, because our old selves became close to us all these years. At times we will miss our addiction, and we have to acknowledge that. But with patience we learn to find new goals for our energies and new aims for our desires. What is ended is a way of life that led us into pain and sorrow and hopelessness. We can let it go now, for it is over and we are on the path of new beginnings.

I mourn and accept the passing of my addicted self, and I welcome the beginning of a new life.

PW

*I lay in a meadow until the unwrinkled serenity
entered in my bones, and made me one with
the still greenery, the drifting clouds.*
— Alice James

Thoughts sometimes whirl in our mind like motes of dust, and our serenity disappears, just like fog in sunshine. Yet nothing is more important to our recovery than serenity; it is at the heart of our ability to be abstinent.

True serenity is inner peace that allows us to view the world realistically. We are involved yet detached at the same time. There can be storms surrounding us, but at the center of ourselves, all is calm.

Serenity depends on many small things. It may feel shaky during times of stress. During those times we can be gentle, patient, and forgiving with ourselves. We must remember how to nurture our serenity. Solitude, soothing music, quiet conversation, nutritious food, prayer, ideas — all can feed our body, mind, emotions, and spirit so that we may thrive. Most important, serenity depends on realizing God's presence in our inner being. Then, no matter what happens, we know all is well.

I can choose to free myself of obstacles to my serenity by nurturing peace within.

SK

Those who love not their fellow-beings live unfruitful lives, and prepare for their old age a miserable grave.
— *Percy Bysshe Shelley*

Sometimes by looking at older people, we get an inkling of how they lived their lives. They may be serene and humorous, surrounded by friends and loved ones. They may be grim and dry, isolated and afraid. By their fruits shall we know them.

If we continue to live deeply in our addiction, our lives will shrink into narrowness and suffocation. There is nothing so constricting as living a life of sex addiction, with its powerlessness, its hopelessness, and its secrecy.

Our programs compel us to take Steps — Steps to increase our spiritual relationship with ourselves, with others, with our Higher Power. We learn to give and take, to offer help to others, and to accept love and friendship in our turn. We come to know a simple truth: we are all wayfarers on a journey whose strongest challenge is the help we can give to others on the journey.

We don't need to run toward a miserable grave. We can walk with dignity along the path of life.

We need to take steps to join in the give-and-take of life.

PW

The search for a new personality is futile; what is fruitful is the human interest the old personality can take in new activities.

— Cesare Tavese

Complete these sentences: For fun, I like to: _____ _____. My favorite color is: _____. Five good things about me are: _____. Hard, isn't it? It's usually easier to come up with five awful things about ourselves. Yet, knowing who we are and being able to state it is a good exercise in self-esteem. It feels good to be able to make positive statements about ourselves. We get a new sense of our identity, especially when we take the risk of telling someone else about ourselves. It's the small things, our preferences and idiosyncrasies, that add color and substance to our personalities.

The longer we're in recovery, the more we enjoy our unique combination of qualities. We can start by affirming them to ourselves often. We can focus on ourselves, not in grandiosity or self-centered ways, but lovingly. Getting to know ourselves is an adventure, one we can enjoy each day.

I am unique. There is only one person like me. I am worthwhile, competent, and lovable.

SK

Childhood is the kingdom where nobody dies.
— *Edna St. Vincent Millay*

Children feel themselves all-powerful in an infinite world. Nothing disappears, nothing passes away. In our earliest days our pleasures were limitless and timeless. Reality was only an obstacle to gratification.

Sex addicts often remain fixed in a similar pleasure-oriented world. We don't like it when someone says no to us. We sometimes try to manipulate reality to suit our own purposes. We may look upon others as objects of gratification. In our fantasies, we often recreate the omnipotent, timeless world of childhood where we are in total control. Our pleasures know no bounds.

We need to remain childlike and full of wonder, but at the same time we must put away these childish fantasies. We can be creative without believing ourselves immortal and invincible. We can return to the kingdom of our earliest days without playing the little despot.

Let's remember the uniqueness of our childhood and leave behind its self-centeredness. Love of others and love of life is the antidote to the narrow circle of our addiction.

Let me remain in touch with my childhood and at the same time expand my experience of the world as it is.

PW

Desire. Desire. The nebula opens
in space, unseen
Your heart utters its great beats
in solitude.

— *Adrienne Rich*

A common fear for newcomers to the program is that they are doomed to never again be sexual. After all, alcoholics and other drug addicts stop drinking and using other drugs. Newcomers often worry that our abstinence is the same. Sex addiction, however, is not like other addictions. We don't put a cork in the bottle and walk away.

Our challenge is to learn how to experience our sexuality within abstinence. We do not want to, nor can we, remove our sexuality. What has to go is the addiction. Once we are abstinent, we begin to see ourselves as whole people, and our sexuality assumes its appropriate place within us. In abstinence, as each of us defines it, we experience safety, respect, and self-esteem. We also find the wondrous connection that comes when we share our sexuality with someone else. We let go of sex as we used to know it and replace it with something far better.

Today, I will experience my abstinence as it is appropriate for me. If I am sexual, I can still be abstinent.

SK

*The essence of a belief is the establishment
of a habit.*

— *Charles Pearce*

Often we may balk at the idea of believing in a Higher
Power because we have been taught to "go it alone" and
not trust in anything or anyone outside ourselves. It is
hard to change beliefs, especially when we are more
or less comfortable with what we have developed over
the years.

To change our beliefs is not simply an intellectual
effort. It comes from discussion and debate and trying
out new behaviors.

That's the value of our Twelve Step group where we
find spiritual nourishment and strength. It is here that
we learn to change our attitudes and develop self-esteem.
As we start to act within our program of recovery, we
find that our beliefs become strengthened when we get
into the habit of thinking in new and positive ways.

---

*By integrating the values of the program into my life, I will
find that these beliefs become mine.*

PW

Even a stopped clock is right twice a day.
— Marie Ebner von Eschenbach

One of the greatest gifts we can give ourselves is for-giveness. When we remember the past, we often find we were much harder on ourselves than we were on other people. We may no longer even remember some of our misdeeds, but it's not so easy to erase the effects of self-punishment on our identity and self-esteem.

There is no need for us to punish ourselves. We can make amends to ourselves just as we do to others. And then we can forgive ourselves, just as we forgive others, and just as we are forgiven by them.

When we find it hard to forgive ourselves and let go, there are actions we can take: We can call someone, work the Tenth Step, or try to find the real feelings beneath the urge to be so hard on ourselves. We can still be honest and choose gentleness. We can also keep our perspective, seeing things realistically and not creat-ing a catastrophe where there is none. We can turn to our Higher Power, asking for a higher forgiveness and be assured of our Higher Power's understanding and love.

Do I have a hidden investment in refusing to forgive myself? I know that forgiving myself is loving myself.

SK

Touch the earth, love the earth, honor the earth, her plains, her valleys, her hills, and her seas; rest your spirit in her solitary places.
— *Henry Beston*

Many of us take life for granted and don't bother to look around and praise the world for its radiance. Especially if we are addicts, we tend to dwell in ourselves and forget that we are part of a world full of mystery and living beauty.

Sex addiction, in particular, cuts us off from contact with the living world. We strive for and crave a pleasure that satisfies only ourselves. That pleasure becomes more and more empty of meaning as we repeat it compulsively. We don't really know what we are looking for, but we know what we find — darkness and despair.

Let's move toward the light, the light of the living world. Whether we go to nature for study or relaxation or adventure or solitude, we can always enhance our world and the world around us through that contact. We come to feel part of something more enduring and more stimulating than our deluded selves, and our lives continue to grow and expand.

I'm learning to look outward, to revel in the simple beauties of the world around me.

PW

All natures are in nature.
                    — Jennie Jerome Churchill

None of us comes into recovery the same. We each have a different story. We may look at our recovering brothers and sisters and compare our lives and recoveries to theirs. We may compare ourselves to those we call "normal." Such comparisons are pointless, however. It's human to look for similarities between ourselves and others; we all search for connection. But it's freeing to realize that each of us is unique.

Some people are healthier than we are, and some people are sicker. Neither state need reflect on us, because each of us is where we're supposed to be — that's the program's wisdom. We can give ourselves credit for our growth by remembering where we started and by acknowledging how far we've come. We can also refuse to live with perfectionistic expectations that lead to discouragement and self-sabotage. There is hope and comfort in knowing that we all have both similarities and differences.

Today, I will accept the differences between myself and others and learn to trust and love them.

SK

> *It is the function of creative people to perceive*
> *the relations between thoughts, or things, or*
> *forms of expression that may seem utterly*
> *different, and to be able to combine them into*
> *some new forms — the power to connect the*
> *seemingly unconnected.*
>
> — William Plomer

When we listen, in our groups, to others speaking of their addiction and their recovery, we may not identify with every part of their story. But if we are attentive to the details, we sense the pattern in lives that are different from our own...and yet strangely familiar.

We are all part of the human family. As we journey forward, our paths change and diverge. And that is healthy. But beyond the splendid range of diversity, our goals are surely similar, as we search for wonder, wisdom, fellowship, and the great adventure of love.

If we talk and listen attentively to others, we will learn about our own lives — our hopes and sorrows, our striving and failure, our courage and despair. Out of this loving exchange will come the signs of our own serenity.

By talking and listening, I have come to see the patterns in others' lives, and I am learning to connect them to my own life and my recovery.

PW

Show us the straight way, the way of those on whom Thou has bestowed Thy Grace, those whose portion is not wrath and who go not astray.

— The Koran

Faith, hope, and love are creative forces. When we learn to live every day in faith, hope, and love, we live in a spiritual place. It is then that the spiritual awakening promised in Step Twelve becomes real. Our spiritual awakening provides the drive, the motivation, the wisdom, and the energy that inspire our stories of recovery.

Faith helps us take the leap: to live in recovery rather than addiction. Hope keeps us alive. It gives us a reason to keep going, especially when things are darkest. And love? For sex addicts, love is the epitome of recovery, the force of goodness restored to us through our sincere willingness to have it again in our lives. Love is the most creative force of all: indefinable, human, divine, powerful. It is our reason to be and to become. When we team love with our faith and hope, we know absolutely that our recovery can take us beyond where we could have ever before dreamed.

Hatred, faithlessness, and despair have no place in my life. Rather, I will feel faith, hope, and love in every part of my being.

SK

They who lose today may win tomorrow.
— *Cervantes*

Sex addiction makes us losers. Our compulsive behavior and our fear of intimacy have made us lose friends, lose touch with our Higher Power, and lose our sense of ourselves. We have fled from intimacy and community and found ourselves in places of shame and isolation.

But in our groups we begin to rediscover ourselves through a new relationship with others and with our Higher Power. We accept that we are part of worlds greater than ourselves, and we tap into the power that comes from love. In doing so we win back our selves.

Winning or losing is not as important in sports or business as it is when our lives are at stake. In sex addiction, our lives *are* at stake: we risk losing everything — family, reputation, friends, jobs, health, sanity, the possibility of intimacy and love. But this doesn't have to happen if we follow our program Step by Step.

Let us resolve to be winners where our own lives are concerned.

We are all winners when we own our sexuality and surround it with intimacy and love.

PW

If you scatter thorns, don't go barefoot.
— *Italian proverb*

When we're feeling, thinking, or behaving negatively, a way to change is to choose its opposite: we can counter dishonesty with honesty, fear with trust, and self-hatred with compassion for ourselves. We can let go of rage by admitting our needs. Rather than resentment, we can choose gratitude.

Developing positive feelings and behavior generates serenity and prepares us for the decision to turn our will over to our Higher Power. It also keeps us in the present, giving us power to make decisions without the preoccupation that comes with negativity.

As we bring ourselves back to the positive during the day, we can do it with gentleness. We will be amazed as positive feelings and actions become alive within us and become our reality.

While taking inventory today, I can list the negative feelings I struggle with and the positive ones that will counteract them.

SK

The absurd man is he who never changes.
— *Auguste Barthélémy*

We often feel sick and tired of being ourselves, because it seems we are always the same, never changing. And this is especially true for sex addicts: our emotional lives often seem like treadmills, never varying in their fantasies and rituals. We haven't acted to alter things; we've only acted out. And in acting out we were driven by a compulsion to repeat actions that gave us little pleasure and no joy.

Sometimes the same feelings come to us in recovery. We say, "Everything's just the same." Or, "I'm just not getting anywhere." Our day-to-day lives seem more or less the same; nothing dramatic has happened, nothing special is going to happen. Inertia. Despair.

Let's look around at others in our group and check things out. We may be able to see more clearly in others the changes that have taken place. Yes, we become aware that John is different, more restful, and Mary is energetic and more outgoing. Change may take place slowly, but it does happen. For sure.

We are changing too. For sure.

Let me become aware of the changes taking place in me each day.

PW

Whom they have injured, they also hate.
— Seneca

When someone has something we want, we may be surprised at the depth and suddenness with which envy can overwhelm us. One moment, we're happy; the next, we're filled with longing. Once we become honest with ourselves and admit we feel envious, we can start to work on ridding ourselves of it. We have uncounted blessings in our lives, and if we simply take the time to count them, envy will fade from our mind as gratitude takes over.

Gratitude can help release envy, especially gratitude for our abstinence today from sex addiction. We can also call a group member to share the feelings underneath the envy. Our challenge in recovery is to accept ourselves as we are and let that be enough. It is, in fact, more than enough because all that we are comes from God. It's better to keep seeing ourselves as the proverbial glass: half-full, not half-empty. We can bless and release whatever person, event, or thing that led to the envy so we may be ourselves, whole, once again.

Envy is obsessive. I will trust in my own path, rather than pouring salt on the wounds of my envy.

SK

I am seeking, I am striving, I am in it with
all my heart.
— *Vincent Van Gogh*

Not only was Van Gogh a stunning artist, he was also a man of intense spiritual energy, living fully for his painting and for others. He loved his work and his life, and he believed that art could change the way we relate to others and to the world.

We all must seek and strive, in order to find what is rich and creative in our lives. If we are addicted to sex without love, our hearts will have become impoverished and empty. We lack spiritual nourishment and the power to give to others. Sex addiction thrives only in the shadow of death.

But luckily there are creative people like Van Gogh who have the power to enrich life not only through their art but through their passion for the adventure of living. They, and others like them, convince us that we owe it to life to get well and find love and truth and beauty that live forever in the heart.

I am grateful that there are creative spirits among us, and
I want to enrich my own life through their example.

PW

A friend is a gift you give yourself.
— *Robert Louis Stevenson*

As sex addicts, we usually want more; we believe more means better. But there are some things where less is more, and one of them is a close friendship. The truth is, we don't have many special friends; that's why they're special.

Between such friends there is a bond of understanding, honesty, acceptance, and love that is valued more over time. Trusted friends offer us the chance to learn to be intimate, to let ourselves be known, time and time again, as we truly are. And from that mutual sharing, we receive what we need. We can take risks, secure in the knowledge that the friendship will stand the test. We don't have to be perfect because we're loved as we are. These relationships possess an innate freedom.

Friendships like these can be platonic or romantic. It doesn't matter. Through good times and bad, we sense our Higher Power's presence completing a divine triangle of growth and love.

Today, I am grateful for my special friends. May my love be a blessing to them, as theirs is to me.

SK

I am the master of my fate
I am the captain of my soul.
— *William Henley*

If we were truly masters of our fate, we would have absolute control over ourselves and have nothing to fear. Illness, old age, or addiction wouldn't threaten us. Indeed we would be superhuman and immortal.

Many of us were brought up to believe that our ego and our will are the most important parts of our lives, and that to fail is intolerable. We did not learn that we are each a part of a universe that includes many things bigger than any one individual — language, other people, culture, nature, and death. All these realities deeply affect our lives, and, in some way, govern and control us.

Our sex addiction has convinced us that we are part of a sick system that includes our addiction. To transcend our addiction, we needed to find another more supportive and inclusive set of behaviors and relationships. We can continue to connect with other people and find a place where we are comfortable and free. In our groups we find such a place; we find people with whom we can relax and develop our new selves.

I am learning to change my attitudes toward fate and control, and I realize that I am part of a whole network of relations with others and with the universe.

Only one who listens can speak.
— *Dag Hammarskjöld*

Inevitably, there will be times when a relationship becomes difficult. Maybe it's a friendship that has conflicts, or a romantic relationship that suddenly, terrifyingly, starts to fall apart.

As addicts, a shaky relationship can trigger our fear of abandonment. That's when we may feel torn between our old, addictive behavior and our recovering behavior. Do we give up and run? Do we hang on, even though we may not want to? How honest should we be? What should be left unsaid, perhaps better shared with someone else? These are only some of the questions we have to ask ourselves.

The wisdom of the program is to do nothing until we know what we want to do. All things, including relationships, are on God's time. Until — or when — we come to a decision, we can live a day at a time, making phone calls, going to meetings, working our program. All we can do is live this moment and give ourselves the love and nurturing we need until the difficulty finally comes to an end. The outcome may not be what we expected, but we can handle that too.

I accept all my relationships as they are today. I will give them my best.

SK

A kleptomaniac can't help helping himself.
— Henry Morgan

Other people's addictions may sometimes strike us as amusing — hiding the bottle of booze in the toilet tank, putting the stolen umbrella down the trouser leg, sneaking a cigarette behind the garage. There is something silly, rigid, and uncompromising about an obsession that causes people to live lives of secrecy and deception. We may laugh at others — but not often enough at ourselves.

Perhaps it will help us to look at ourselves and laugh a little as we search frenziedly for the picture or image or object or person or ritual we crave. How selfish and yet how comic we are when we narrow our vision to follow only our own degraded and self-serving desires!

Laughter may help to bring us back to sanity and humanity. In the theater when we laugh with others, we feel a part of the human community. Laughter, that very human form of expression, integrates and heals.

I am developing a sense of humor that helps me see myself in a new way.

PW

Desire realized is sweet to the soul.
— *Prov. 13:19*

If we were deprived as children, we may still live with an emptiness inside. Of what were we deprived? Love, security, validation, acceptance, caring, compassion? We compensated by learning to bear the deprivation and survive. As adults, we're still surviving. We settle; we don't ask for things because we believe we don't deserve anything. But making do with life's crumbs leads to resentment, self-pity, and feeling deprived. We remain children, instead of becoming adults who feel competent and worthwhile.

There is a balance between wanting nothing and wanting everything. If we can broaden our thinking to include such words as plenty, fulfillment, pleasure, and satisfaction, we will start to believe there is enough of everything. It is then we become aware of the fullness of life around and within us. Living in the present helps us realize we have everything we need in this moment. That realization helps us feel worthwhile, competent — and fulfilled.

God, please take away my fear of satisfaction and pleasure. Grant me an awareness of how good life is, whether or not it brings me what I expect.

SK

Pain is the root of knowledge.
>   — Simone Weil

Many of us still fear pain and flee its onset. In the past, we did almost anything to avoid being hurt, and we were unwilling to take risks with our emotional life. We sought pleasure in what we considered the safety of our addiction, though deep down we knew we were playing a dangerous game with our sanity. But at least we wouldn't make ourselves vulnerable — or so we thought.

Life without pain is an impossibility. And the same is true of love. Our loved ones may grow away from us for a while. They may fall sick, leave us, or die. We cannot control life. Accepting it and loving it as it is, with everything that is unpredictable and painful about it, is one of the greatest challenges of recovery.

We can accept pain as a part of life, even as a part of our growth and health. We can accept pain when we have a foundation of serenity gained through our program — the serenity to accept the things we cannot change. We give up the false sense of power that results from closing ourselves off from pain, and, at last, we feel fully alive.

I want to come to terms with suffering and pain and live life with courage, and, ultimately, with serenity in my heart.

PW

Celebration is a forgetting in order to remember.
A forgetting of ego, of problems, of difficulties.
A letting go.

— Matthew Fox

Holidays can be a real test of recovery, particularly for those of us who still struggle with sex addiction on a day-to-day basis. It's especially hard for those of us who are alone.

It is a time to take good care of ourselves. We can go to extra meetings, keep up with phone calls and try to be honest, rather than jolly. We can refuse to lose ourselves in sex, drinking, or overeating. We can find other recovering people to be with.

Perhaps holidays offer us the chance to reflect on the impact our addiction has had on our relationships and how much sharing these special times with others means. We are also able to appreciate what we already have, to better recognize our blessings because we have known the pain and deprivation of our illness.

The program is ours this holiday season, offering us peace, simplicity, and reality. We can choose an attitude of hope and gratitude. In letting go of expectations, we may find much more to celebrate than we anticipated.

I have enough, I do enough, I am enough.

SK

To eat bread without hope is still slowly to starve to death.

— *Pearl S. Buck*

If we exist without hope we will surely lose our hold on life. Those of us addicted to sexual behavior without love or intimacy move step-by-step into despair. We retreat into our little worlds of selfish gratification. Gradually, we forget what it means to be truly alive.

If we look around at people in recovery, we are struck by the sparkle in their eyes, the color in their cheeks, the spring in their step. They have come back to life. They have learned how to care again and to be unafraid of closeness. They have found life again in all its vibrancy and promise of change and renewal.

This kind of energy is contagious, and forms one of the many advantages of working together in a group. We see people change and come back to life. We learn how lonely they were when they sought only their own sexual pleasure. Their recovery touches our lives and inspires us to come back out of the darkness of our addiction into the clear light of day.

My life is changed through contact with others in recovery.

PW

All truth passes through three stages. First, it is ridiculed. Second, it is violently opposed. Third, it is accepted as being self-evident.
— *Arthur Schopenhauer*

Contrary to popular belief, there is no such thing as a "typical" sex addict. We are told that the typical addict is one sex (male), had one kind of childhood (bad), started engaging in sexual activities (masturbating) and went on to other, more reprehensible actions (molestation and mayhem). The truth is each of our stories is unique and belongs only to us.

We are male and female. We are married, single, heterosexual, homosexual. We have used pornography, had affairs, fantasized, cruised, abused our sexuality, and broken the law. We have also wept, lived in silent fear, felt shame, suffered remorse, and agonized over our powerlessness. Now we have a name for what we've experienced: sex addiction.

Our fellowship comes from our common suffering as well as our common experience, strength, and hope. Society may not understand our addiction, but we do and there are more of us growing and loving in recovery every day.

There is power in accepting reality. I can accept the reality of my addiction and find recovery.

SK

While there is a soul in prison, I am not free.
— *Eugene V. Debs*

One of our missions in recovery is to carry the message of our program to other sex addicts. We believe we have an obligation to spread the notion of community and caring as widely as possible.

For some of us this is difficult. When we go out to introduce someone to the program, we probably feel shy and embarrassed at first; in our culture it is hard to talk openly about sex addiction. Yet, as we gain confidence in the program and in ourselves, we find it easier to talk to strangers and spread the word. Talking to others in this way increases our sense of connecting with the human community. We also become freer in helping others rid themselves of their addiction.

We are all related to one another in our loneliness and our pain. And as long as there are people suffering from the disease of sex addiction, we are all deeply affected. We must do what we can to help.

I am proud to talk openly about my addiction and help those who also suffer from it.

PW

One is as one is, and the love that can't encompass both is a poor sort of love.
— Marya Mannes

All of us have struggled to find the best way to forgive ourselves and others. Forgiving isn't easy. In fact, when we've been deeply hurt or victimized by someone else, we may feel we can't forgive. Yet, for our own peace of mind and in order to let go, we may finally try. It's been suggested that forgiveness is easier under certain conditions: a positive connection with the person we want to forgive, a deep relationship with God as we understand God, and lots of time.

Forgiveness is often preceded by grieving fully; we must first heal from the harm that was done to us. In their honesty, power, and wisdom, the Twelve Steps lead us gently through the process of forgiving ourselves and others. Many of us have also experienced our Higher Power's unconditional forgiveness, which gives us a model. We acknowledge our responsibility for our actions, we let go of resentment, we grieve, and, finally, we forgive.

Today, I will Let Go and Let God.

SK

We are here and it is now. Further than that,
all knowledge is moonshine.
— *H. L. Mencken*

Some us may think it's selfish to be too concerned with the present. Shouldn't we be thinking lofty thoughts or planning for the future? And the past — don't we have to get it in perspective?

There's good sense in all that. But let's remember we don't live in the past or the future. We do have painful memories and they are a real part of our present. But only a part, so that we don't have to obsessively fill our present with the past to acknowledge our history. We aren't there; we're here. It's not then, it's now, and always will be.

Learning to live in the here and now is a way of centering ourselves and bringing the world and other people into focus. If we experience fully what's happening at every moment, our lives will expand and deepen and become enriched by a vivid sense of being truly alive.

I don't want to spend my life wishing things were different.
I am content to be who I am, where I am, now.

PW

Faith and doubt both are needed — not as antagonists, but working side by side to take us around the unknown curve.

— Lillian Smith

When we pray the Serenity Prayer and ask God to grant us the serenity to accept the things we cannot change, we immediately and humbly admit that our willpower and ego are, in the end, powerless over certain realities. There are innumerable things we can't change, including our addiction to sex, other people, inflation, what time the paper is delivered, and the price of milk.

It's simpler just to accept that we're not in control. Then, we can turn our energy to something more productive — like changing the things we can. In the end, these are usually things about ourselves we don't like, which is why change takes so much courage. In the Serenity Prayer, we're not asking for control. Control has no place in our lives now that we're in recovery. Rather, we need to try to put aside our fear, which is usually behind our need to control. Then, we can move on, realizing that serenity, courage, and wisdom are gifts from God.

I will never outgrow the Serenity Prayer; I always need serenity, courage, and wisdom.

SK

An idealist is one who, on noticing that a rose smells better than a cabbage, concludes that it will also make better soup.
— H. L. Mencken

We are often justly proud of our ideals as we attempt to live by them in our daily lives. Ideals give us hope and help us dream of better worlds. But ideals can easily turn into doctrines and become rigid. They can cause us to shun diversity so that we make false assumptions. The humble cabbage may not fill our ideal of beauty, but it can be transformed into an excellent soup.

Many of us sex addicts are perfectionists who have been brought up to believe in nothing other than the ideal. When we fall away from perfection, we plunge from the heights of idealism to the depths of misery and self-abuse.

We can do better by being less perfectionistic. When we reveal and accept our real strengths and defects with Steps Four and Five, and humbly turn them over in Six and Seven, we get a new perspective on ourselves and a true sense of balance. We learn to be flexible and to appreciate the diversity of life (even the humble cabbage).

Even if I don't especially like cabbage soup, I can recognize that all things may be good to those who love life and keep their eyes wide open.

THE TWELVE STEPS OF ALCOHOLICS ANONYMOUS*

1. We admitted we were powerless over alcohol—that our lives had become unmanageable.
2. Came to believe that a Power greater than ourselves could restore us to sanity.
3. Made a decision to turn our will and our lives over to the care of God *as we understood Him.*
4. Made a searching and fearless moral inventory of ourselves.
5. Admitted to God, to ourselves, and to another human being the exact nature of our wrongs.
6. Were entirely ready to have God remove all these defects of character.
7. Humbly asked Him to remove our shortcomings.
8. Made a list of all persons we had harmed, and became willing to make amends to them all.
9. Made direct amends to such people wherever possible, except when to do so would injure them or others.
10. Continued to take personal inventory and when we were wrong promply admitted it.
11. Sought through prayer and meditation to improve our conscious contact with God *as we understood Him,* praying only for knowledge of His will for us and the power to carry that out.
12. Having had a spiritual awakening as the result of these steps, we tried to carry this message to alcoholics, and to practice these principles in all our affairs.

---

*The Twelve Steps are taken from *Alcoholics Anonymous* (Third Edition), published by AA World Services, Inc., New York, N.Y., 59-60. Reprinted with permission.

INDEX

Other meditation books that will interest you . . .

Each Day a New Beginning
Daily Meditations for Women

The first daily meditation guide created by and for women involved in Twelve Step recovery programs. Hundreds of thousands of women have found help in this collection of thoughts and reflections that offer hope, strength, and guidance every day of the year. 400 pp.
Order No. 1076

Touchstones
A Book of Daily Meditations for Men

Created especially for men in recovery, this daily meditation guide offers insight into emotions, becoming whole people, finding spiritual enlightenment, masculinity, anger, communication and sexuality, among many other topics. *Touchstones* possesses a rare blend of inspiration and contemplation that will touch any man involved in a Twelve Step program. 400 pp.
Order No. 5029
